Finding the
Healer Within

Finding the Healer Within

Beth Moran, RN, CNP
with
Kathy Schultz

NLN Press • New York
Pub. No. 14-6819

Copyright © 1996
National League for Nursing
350 Hudson Street, New York, NY 10014

The views expressed in this book reflect those of the authors and do not necessarily reflect the official views of the National League for Nursing.

Library of Congress Cataloging-in-Publication Data

Moran, Beth.
    Finding the healer within / Beth Moran with Kathy Schultz.
        p.   cm.
    "Pub. no. 14-6819."
    Includes bibliographical references and index.
    ISBN 0-88737-681-9
    1. Women—Health and hygiene.   2. Psychoneuroimmunology.
3. Holistic nursing.   4. Nurse practitioners.   I. Schultz, Kathy,
1948–   . II. Title.
    [DNLM: 1. Women's Health Services.   2. Holistic Nursing.   3. Nurse
Practitioners.   WA 309 M829F 1996]
    RA778.M758   1996
    613'.04244—dc20
    DNLM/DLC
                                                                                    96-5862
                                                                                    CIP

This book was set in Caledonia by Publications Development Company, Crockett, Texas. The editor was Allan Graubard. The printer was Book Crafters. The cover was designed by Lauren Stevens.

Printed in the United States of America

*The concept of teacher as student
and student as teacher
is not new.
It has been spoken of by the wise souls
of every generation.
There is much learning
to be derived from the teaching process.
But the teacher must remain the student
if the teacher is to grow.*

From Emmanuel's Book

Foreword

Nurses are practical, observant people who often pick up what physicians may overlook. While medicine often looks at the body as an assembly of various parts, nursing has always been based on a whole person approach. Not only do we have bodies, but we are emotional and spiritual beings as well. When emotions are blocked or people feel helpless and trapped, they often fall ill and may get worse despite the finest treatment. On the other hand, when people feel worthwhile, connected to others, and in harmony with life, they tend to stay well. If they do become ill, such stress-hardy optimistic people often improve even when medical treatment for their condition is not expected to help.

The observational wisdom of nursing has been validated scientifically during the past two decades with the advent of a new field of medical research called psychoneuroimmunology, or PNI. Research indicates that emotions are the link between mind and body. Beth Moran explores this exciting new field and suggests simple, practical strategies of healing that can sometimes reverse illness naturally, and can always help mobilize the body's defenses to cooperate in the best way with medical treatment. The hope is that all of us can develop the attitudes and lifestyles that are consistent with improved health, and most importantly with creative, peaceful, joyful lives.

JOAN BORYSENKO, PhD

Preface

As dawn breaks on the twenty-first century, women's health care will see many changes. Contemporary women give vigorous voice to concerns about health care and healing, and particularly about the "healers" to whom they entrust themselves. Responsible health care practitioners are coming to understand that "responsible" means being answerable to the female patient whose life is at stake.

I am a nurse practitioner, and I provide women's health care services with a holistic emphasis. I am unceasingly inspired by physicians who are well-known for their holistic approach to medicine. Dr. Christiane Northrup, Dr. Andrew Weil, Dr. Bernie Siegel, and many physicians in my own community have, over the years, embodied the spirit and philosophy of holistic healing. I know there are many other physicians, worldwide, who are practicing holistic medicine as well. Despite this gradually occuring shift in philosophy, I am constantly surprised by the number of patients who tell me they are more comfortable with nurses than with doctors. It makes a difference to know they are in the hands of someone who is concerned as much with their symptoms as with their selves.

Cost is a weighty matter to consumers of health care, especially in these times when they are scrutinizing what they pay practitioners, and why they are being asked to pay it. A woman should want to know why costly tests and procedures are required, and whether they will benefit her. The marvels of modern (and costly) technology notwithstanding, are there alternative options?

Some nurse practitioners are starting to ask the same question. Whether this question is asked by consumers, doctors, or nurses, the goal is the same—to effect changes in the patient's interest and for the patient's good health.

In this book, I have attempted to answer some of the questions women are asking, and to inspire the reader to become more inquisitive and inventive about the *healing* process itself. During the process of writing, I realized the impracticality of describing the plethora of fine research that has been conducted for many years in the various areas of healing, so I have provided an extensive bibliography which I hope encourages readers to become their own investigators, and to seek out information that will help them find their own healer within. On a continuing basis, women need to become informed consumers of health care and to understand that every day new research, new information, new treatments, and new products become available. The number of choices available to us is constantly growing.

Many, many factors, in addition to what we professionals learn about in chemistry and anatomy class, contribute to the healing process. We can find out what they are if we listen to our bodies. I believe our bodies tell us everything we need to know about ourselves, and that healing is a process that requires as much from the patient as from the practitioner. Symptoms are not the cause, but the effect. From the holistic perspective, illness has as much to do with how we live our lives as it does with the presence of a germ. We all have a healer within us. My job as a nurse practitioner is to help people find that healer within.

BETH MORAN, RN, CNP

Sag Harbor, New York
March, 1996

Acknowledgments

I would like to thank all of the physicians who have collaborated with me over the years to make my practice possible. Dr. Aaron David was the first to encourage me, and to extol the virtues of a nurse practitioner practice. Dr. Wilfrido Dianzon was a supportive and non-judgmental collaborator who expected nothing in return. Dr. Mary Zachary is a role model for women, and for holistic primary caregivers. She agreed to collaborate with my associate and me because she supports and believes in the goals of our holistic nurse practitioner practice.

My associate Linda Coleman has stood beside me night and day, and her unswerving support for our practice sustains me. I would like to thank my assistant, Laurie Frick, for her tireless typing, and especially for her help in administering the office during my absences, so that I could write. I would also like to thank Dr. John Bishop for his assistance and for his long-time support.

I am so grateful to all the people who encouraged me to write this book, especially my friend, Joan Fitzgerald, who said I must write it. Rich MacArthur saw it happening long before I did and has supported and encouraged me through every step, through both disappointment and excitement. A special thanks to Nancy Nelson, who came to me as a client and told me she knew I thought I had nothing to say, but that she thought I had a lot to say, and I should say it before someone else does. Once I began writing, Niro Markoff Asistent, in her steady and gracious way, encouraged me to press on whenever setbacks overwhelmed me.

I am grateful to all of my friends in AA and AlAnon who have listened to me and helped me to find spiritual guidance and my inner voice. A humble thanks goes to all of my patients. They validated me, and taught me so many things I never learned in school or from a textbook. A lot of gratitude goes to my mother, Virginia Metzler, a wonderful writer who never found her voice, but helped me to find mine.

A great deal of my work was inspired by my grandmother, Virginia Breunich, who taught me about unconditional love and forgiveness, and by my dad, Laurent Metzler, whose kindness and quiet guidance led to me having my own practice and speaking my truth.

Last, a huge thank you to my co-writer, Kathy Schultz, without whose insight, fortitude, love, and encouragement this would never have happened, and to our editor, Allan Graubard, whose excitement and sensitivity brought this book to fruition.

B.M.

Contents

—1—

The Nurse Practitioner and You

For over a week now, Kim had felt the kind of stomach pain that breeds frightful possibilities. Was it an infection? Was she pregnant? Or could it be the fearsome ovarian cancer?

"Will I like this new doctor?" she wondered, almost aloud, as she entered the waiting room of an unknown practitioner. He had been highly recommended, but still her nerves churned. Will it be okay? What will the answers to my questions be? Sweat drizzled down her hands. Wedged between two other patients on an icy chrome chair, her back against a white wall, she waited. Her appointed hour came and passed. Fifteen more minutes ticked by, plenty of time for all sorts of anxious thoughts to clog her mind. She wished she was home in front of the fireplace, petting her dogs.

Finally Kim heard her name. She was escorted into an exam room, asked to undress and put on a gown. Obediently she changed, and then waited another seemingly eternal ten minutes.

The doctor walked in, introduced himself, and asked why she had come. He seemed preoccupied and rushed, as if he were trying to balance many balls in the air at once. As he performed an entire physical and a pelvic exam, she stared up at the ceiling floodlights. He said he would have her test results back in a week. Just then, a second assistant popped in and asked him to come to the phone—another patient had gone into labor. Kim realized how busy he must be, but somehow she felt cheated. Unsettled, detached and disconnected, she got dressed. There must be a more comforting way to do this.

The bright lights and medicinal smells had intimidated her, and she had forgotten to ask her questions. Now she would just have to wait for the test results. Perhaps she could ask the secretary or the nurse. The doctor was polite, but obviously overworked. She had some ideas about how she would have preferred this to happen, but she knew she could not change the system. She wished she had spoken up instead of clamming up. Where was her voice when she needed it? Why did these situations always prove so scary and demeaning? She hated medical offices and vowed she would avoid them as much as possible.

I first noticed this ever-widening gap between patient and health care provider thirty years ago when I trained as a registered nurse (RN) at Pennsylvania Hospital in Philadelphia. Working on hospital floors and then later in surgery, I saw that physicians frequently had to be in surgery or involved in the care of critically ill patients, so they could rarely be at the bedside, as we nurses were. In my capacity as a nursing student, I was taught to ask questions about patients' psychosocial history: What were their relationships like? What was their work? How were they functioning as a social being in the world? They were not to be regarded as just No. 32 with a gallbladder or a heart attack. These were issues physicians had no time to address, but when they asked a nurse how a patient was progressing, I could give a thorough answer because I was trained to make fine-grained observations, and to sense changes above and beyond a blood cell count.

One of my later jobs was explaining to patients, pre- and post-operatively, what was happening to their bodies. As a nurse, I had ample time to witness the staggering role fear plays in illness and recovery. Without a nurse to act as buffer between the person and the surgical doctor, patients might have left and never returned, or survived the medical experience with far more fear and anxiety than necessary.

I eventually went back to school to earn a degree in Business Administration, and then became a Patient Advocate in Administration at The New York Hospital. In that position, I worked with patients who were refusing treatments and assisted them in demanding their rights to do so. Part of my job was to investigate complaints and decide whether or not they were valid. I was often charged with managing mismanagement, as every potential lawsuit had to be reviewed and assessed. In the midst of this, I developed a life-threatening melanoma, a type of cancer.

At the time, I had a great deal of unhappiness in my personal life, and the threat of cancer finally pushed me to leave my pressure-cooker marriage. But I felt like I wasn't accomplishing anything in my work either. I intuitively felt that all these factors contributed to my illness. All I was doing was listening to people complain all day long about how they didn't like the hospital, they didn't like the doctors, they didn't like the fruit on the breakfast tray or the beans at lunch, and they were going to sue. My cancer was ultimately treatable, but the experience made me see I was spiritually unsuited for this type of work. I missed being a nurse and caring for people, which was what I had been so drawn to when I chose my career in health care. I returned to school again, this time to become a Certified Nurse Practitioner (CNP).

I was inspired by Margaret Sanger's life and work. Like her, I wanted to make a commitment to give women information, so they would have choices in their lives. I studied at the Margaret Sanger Center in New York City and became a Women's Health Care Nurse Practitioner. In the process, I learned a great deal about both Western and holistic medicine.

After becoming a CNP, I opened my own nursing practice, specializing in women's health care. My practice is holistic because I combine conventional and alternative approaches to medicine. I utilize both traditional Eastern techniques and Western health care. "Western" here means that I apply everything I learned in modern medical hospitals, including prescribing pharmaceutical drugs in accordance with my standards of practice, X-rays, and/or laboratory tests when needed. "Eastern" means that I might also suggest acupuncture, herbal therapy, homeopathy, massage, Rolfing, Reiki, nutritional or psychological counseling if it might alleviate symptoms. A holistic philosophy means that I base assessments more on what patients tell me than on laboratory test results, *because I believe the body tells you everything you need to know.*

The term "holistic" is derived from the word "whole," and it means that a patient is treated as a whole person, rather than treating one symptom as if it were completely isolated from the rest of the body. When women come to me, they are not just a uterus with a Pap smear. They are people who have lives, children, relationships, jobs, exercise routines, spiritual beliefs, and eating habits, *and all these factors impact on their health.* When someone comes to me with a recurrent infection, I don't believe the infection alone is what I'm supposed to look at. I talk to them about what else is happening. What are their stressors? What are their relationships like? Do they exercise? What do they eat? What do they believe in spiritually?

This type of assessment provides clues about the infection. How to stay well in the first place is what I teach people, because it is not my goal to persuade hordes of patients to make multiple office visits. Unnecessary visits or tests cost money, so I avoid that whenever possible. I teach people to take responsibility for themselves in their health care (not needing care is ultimately the biggest money-saver). As a nurse, I had learned to talk and touch, rather than test and treat, and to help patients find their own answers. Early in my training, I was taught to "listen to the patient—she will give you the diagnosis."

I refer patients to nearby physicians, surgeons, or specialists when treatment beyond the scope of my training is required, and I encourage them to make choices based on coherent information. I have developed solid working relationships with many local physicians, so I can refer patients to them and call them with questions when problems beyond my experience arise.

Although nurse practitioners do many of the same things physicians do—prescribe medications, perform examinations, blood pressure measurements, and tests—there are unmistakable differences between a nursing practice and a physician's practice. Patients tell me, "You listen to me. You take time with me and ask me questions. You ask what no doctor has ever asked before." I don't have to make rounds in the hospital or perform surgery or deliver babies, so I am able to spend extra time with people. *The current system is not the fault of physicians; it is the logical end result of a national health care system wherein most doctors are too busy practicing crisis medicine to talk to patients.* They are overwhelmed by how much work they have to do, how many people they have to see, and the life-and-death responsibility that is repeatedly placed on their shoulders. Patients, hospital administrators, and insurance companies are constantly turning to them for answers to life-threatening problems. This is the "Illness Model" of health care. In my practice, I operate from a "Wellness Model."

Central to the Wellness Model is "primary care," which means performing check-ups, treating minor complaints, and helping people find the right physician to treat more serious conditions. But again, my main job is teaching people how to stay well in the first place. *This takes time. There is no quick way to do it.* Sometimes a patient comes to me asking why they were given a certain medication by a physician, or why a certain treatment was recommended. I review with them the anatomy and physiology that could create the illness, as well as the pros and cons of possible treatment. What there is no time for in conventional practice is the very essence of mine.

Over the years, I have learned not to make decisions for patients. People often go to health care providers expecting all the answers, but I allow people to take responsibility for themselves. I encourage them to decide what to do based on their own intuition, and especially their intuition about *what works for them.* When I began my career I thought I had to have all the answers, and for a time I did think I had all the answers. Counterposed to this presumption—for now I understand it as such—was, again, the lesson of nursing school: "Listen to the patients. They will give you the diagnosis." In some physicians' offices there may not be enough time to sit and listen. Physicians can be rushed by practicing high-tech medicine, or they're practicing defensive medicine and feel compelled to order a great number of tests before recommending surgery or medication.

My patients tell me what they want and what they don't want, and this is another difference between a nursing practice and a physician's practice; I am a partner with the patient rather than an authority figure. Nor am I threatened any longer by a patient who says, "No, I don't want that treatment." I have come to believe there are many ways to heal people. Often the conventional combined with a holistic treatment works well. Sometimes modern conventional technique alone is sufficient, and sometimes the holistic alone is all that's needed. I encourage patients to be their own advocates, to scour the library for everything they can find about their illness, to get another opinion, to talk to other people who have had similar illnesses, and to seek out alternative methods that might help them.

My first-time patients are almost always struck by this perception as well: my office does not look like a physician's office. Some research suggests that certain colors are healing in their effect, whereas others are not, and that hospitals and clinics should be painted and decorated in such a way as to promote healing rather than fear. In my office there is no white, starched, chrome motif. Instead, the office and exam room are painted in soft mauve, and decorated with pastel flowered fabrics. Cloth potholders cover the stirrups to protect patients' feet from the cold metal, and the rooms look like rooms in my home. I have attempted to make the environment appear as nonthreatening and nonmedical as possible. This can be done while maintaining antiseptic cleanliness, despite all kinds of arguments to the contrary. Women frequently tell me, "I've never seen an office like this before. It's so relaxed." It overlooks the water and we have soothing music playing quietly. Patients tell me they are afraid of doctors, and some tell me they have not been examined for ten years because of fear. People tell me this happens because they feel doctors talk down to them or don't have time for them, but sometimes these fears are further aggravated by the forbidding environment found in so many hospitals, offices, and clinics, and perpetuated in the name of sanitation. I try to address all of the senses (i.e., visual, auditory, and spiritual) and to create an environment that is safe and welcoming.

Many of our patients cannot be reimbursed for our services by their health care insurance. Iniquitous?—yes, and so it prevails. Some insurance companies reimburse only when a CNP works in a physician's office but not when they have their own independent practice. Patients come to us anyway and pay us out of their own pockets because they feel more relaxed and not so scared.

And what of the role of the nurse practitioner in the twenty-first century? As now, the nurse practitioner will continue to bridge the gap between patient and health care provider, to see the patient as a human being. We nurses have provided and will continue to provide primary care in a nonthreatening, caring fashion. Nurses are taught to educate and listen to patients, and to assess their conditions based on observations as well as clinical data.

I always consider myself a nurse first and a nurse practitioner second. I consider it part of my job to build bridges between nurse practitioners, nurses, and doctors. Nurse practitioners provide a different aspect of health care than physicians, and that does not mean they replace physicians. Rather, we provide service that many physicians are unable to provide. Nurse practitioners, physicians, nurses, nutritionists, and many other technicians together form a team whose goal is the patient's greater good. Many physicians are supportive of the role of the nurse practitioner in private practice, and see us as a valuable member of the health care team. The key word here is *communication*. As nurses we are taught to communicate with patients and with doctors, and to refer patients to physicians when situations beyond our expertise arise. This point often needs clarification in the public's perception of nurse practitioners.

A nursing practice is in some ways more of a teaching practice than anything else, and in this context nurse practitioners are just one arm of a health care team that is sorely needed in many areas. Nursing practices are places where clients can come to ask questions, get information, sort things out, and then take all this information to a physician if needed. We can and most often do make the physician's job easier by saving time he or she doesn't have. Clients tell me they feel more relaxed and more like an "equal," and that they can make much better decisions under these conditions.

I tell women to listen to their bodies, because our bodies tell us everything we need to know to get well. My nursing practice is also a place where people come to learn how to listen to their intuition. As a nurse, I encourage this. So as you read this book, remember—listen to yourself. *You* have all the answers to find the healer within.

—2—

The Mind–Body
Connection
(Psychoneuroimmunology)

Almost every day, I find myself telling patients, "Listen to yourself. Listen to your body. If you listen to what your body is telling you, you will know what is wrong." This approach to health care is often dismissed as irresponsible, because it has not been awash in "scientific proof." Now, however, proof emerges from medical journals in a steady stream. Recent research has revealed how the immune system and the nervous system communicate with each other. So when something upsets you, your immune system feels it, too. The study of this connection is called Psychoneuroimmunology (PNI), known in the vernacular as the Mind-Body Connection. The focus of PNI is how the Neurological System (mind and nerves) is connected to the Immune System.

You may have already thought about the relationship between the mind and the body, and you may have some beliefs about it, especially if you have ever become physically ill over the problems of life.

Margaret Kemeny, a psychologist, and George Solomon, a psychiatrist, both at UCLA, are respected researchers in the field of psychoneuroimmunology.[1] Their research demonstrates that the nervous system and the immune system communicate in a bidirectional fashion. They send chemical messages to one another.

One of Dr. Solomon's findings occurred not in his laboratory, but rather as he was having his shoes shined. He noticed that the shoeshiner's hand was shaking. Solomon asked, "Why is your hand shaking?" The man replied, "Well, I'm 97." A surprised Dr. Solomon inquired, "Why are you still shining shoes at 97?" "Well," the shoeshiner replied, "They're having a 100th birthday party for me in three years. If I don't shine shoes, I will die and I want to be alive for this party. It will be a great party." This corroborated what Solomon had been observing consistently in older, healthy people. He was finding that when people had goals, things to look forward to, their immune systems were strengthened, because if the immune system is talking to the nervous system, what do you think it is saying? "Keep fighting and be strong, because I don't want to miss this great party."

Sometimes a "cure" resembles a miracle. Consider the case of a man I know who was diagnosed with pancreatic cancer and given two months to live. He decided that since he had always wanted to play in a band, he was going to join a band for his last two months of life. He had always been too busy working to do it before. He started playing his clarinet. A year later, he was still playing clarinet in the band. How do we explain that? These are the kinds of cases for which we have no formula in traditional medicine. Medical textbooks refer to them as "spontaneous remissions." Non-medical people call them miracles. I believe such cures are examples of the Mind-Body Connection. We ought not discount the Mind-Body Connection, particularly in the case of so-called "miracles." Joy, contentment, satisfaction, having goals, work or hobbies that we love can keep us alive, and this is no longer an inexplicable mystery. It is a fact that can be scientifically demonstrated by comparing the blood chemistry of fatalistic people to that of optimistic people.

My Own Experience

My own interest in how thinking affects health began a number of years ago when I developed melanoma, a skin cancer that could have metastasized (spread) and killed me. Fear over-whelmed me. I looked at my life and realized I was not happy with certain aspects of it. I was not making a difference in the world, and at one time that had been a goal of mine. I was drinking, smoking, and not happy in my work or my marriage. I decided to change my whole life. I ended my marriage, went back to school, and became a Nurse Practitioner. I opened my own practice, stopped drinking and smoking, started eating well, and exercising.

And most important of all, I began to have fun and live, to take risks and do all the things I had always wanted to do.

I didn't do all of this in the first month, however. That first month I was depressed, and I decided that I was going to die. That was when I decided to change and learn how to live.

I had been working with cancer patients for five years at the time, and I began to feel that there must be a different way to look at illness. Was it just simply that you get sick, you have surgery, you have chemotherapy, you have radiation, and that's it? I felt there must be something more to it than that. I began reading about psychology and nutrition, and their relation to illness. I began my own informal research about why some people got sicker while others got better. I began reading about psychoneuroimmunology.

What the Research Tells Us

We are all exposed to many potential dangers and we all respond to them differently. Why? This is central to PNI. Why does one person get sick and not another? Why is one person able to fight disease and another person is not? It's not just "co-incidence."

There are numerous reasons why people get sick. Sometimes we get sick because of poor nutrition, smoking, excessive alcohol, environmental toxins, genetic predispositions, age, inappropriate medications, stress, past traumas, or unexpressed emotions. All of these can contribute to disease and illness. Medical researchers have studied people who have "elevated" immune responses, such as people who have been HIV positive and well for a very long time, or elderly people who have been well for a long time.[2] By "elevated" we mean that the immune system seems to be working exceptionally well. The general finding was that people who are fatalistic, or who just give up, do not do as well as those who are optimistic, and who look upon their lives as a challenge. It seems to me that "challenge" shifts us into "fighting" mode, causing the immune system to accelerate.

In a study where two laboratory "fighter mice" were locked in a cage together, one mouse eventually seemed to stop fighting and give up.[3] It was examined for immune system functioning, which means the researchers counted and analyzed the mouse's white blood cells in various ways. The "defeated" mouse exhibited what scientists call a suppressed immune system. The other mouse, who had never given up fighting, exhibited an elevated immune response. Kemeny suggests that we have all been "bitten" by life, and we have all been in cages of sorts, and that those of us who choose to fight will have elevated immune responses. Sometimes it is important to fight for what we want. Think back to a time when you stood up for what you wanted, no matter how small or trivial the issue was. Many of us can recall a sense of *physical* well-being, even though the issue may have seemed to be *intellectual* or *emotional.*

Let's look at health care in this connection.

We are now beginning to see people who fight for what they want in their health care. These people, as we might expect, have elevated immune responses. Solomon cites the case of two chemotherapy patients. One patient said to the doctor, "I'm grateful that you will see me, I'm grateful that I can have this therapy, and I really want to do this." The other patient said, "Wait a minute. Why am I having this therapy? What are the risks? What are the benefits? Do I really want to do this? What is it going to cost? Is it going to cure me? Let me think about it." Which responded better to treatment? The answer is clear: The second patient did. Patients who are considered the most "difficult" for doctors to deal with—those with that fighter response—often fare better. I have observed this same thing over and over in my work. It seems that the fighting response somehow causes the immune system to roar into action—and that the mouse experiment is replicated in the human arena every day.

Deepak Chopra, a medical doctor who has conducted research in this field, contends that body cells store everything that we have ever experienced in life, and that everything the mind is unable to express is stored in the body.[4] Part of his theory is that in the gap between body and mind is the spirit, and we need to heal the spirit because it programs the mind. We need to listen to our bodies to figure out just how to heal the spirit. That is something I encourage all my patients to do. Our bodies talk to us in numerous ways, and if we get sick, it is not necessarily a punishment, but rather, a message. Instead of thinking of illness as a punishment for not doing something, it might be more productive to ask, "What is my body saying to me? What do I need to address? What do I need to look at? What do I need to change in my life?"

When we get the news that we have a medical problem, it is important that we not berate ourselves for not practicing positive thinking, or feel guilty by thinking that we caused our illness. This is *not* the time to say, "This is all my fault because I didn't relax and handle my stress well enough." We have all weathered situations that are too stressful to manage easily. It is crucial to the healing process that we be kind to ourselves. PNI is not meant to be used as a weapon with which we kick ourselves when we're down. To do so misses the point.

If we listen to our bodies, we can then try to understand what our bodies are telling us. When we can use pain as a warning, we ask ourselves, "What is going on here? What do I really need to see here?" This is more fruitful than saying, "Oh no, I'm sick and I'm going to die," or "Why did God do this to me?" It is to our advantage to maintain an optimistic perspective (when that is realistically possible), and to be open to what we might be able to learn from our bodies' messages. Illness is an opportunity to grow and change, to heal with the past, to learn to live, and to embrace what we really want.

Numerous studies have documented the effects of placebo (fake) drugs on people's expectations.[5] Typically, half of a group of symptomatic people in a study are given a drug to treat their condition, while the other half are given a placebo which looks exactly like the real drug (pill or liquid). The participants are not told which they're getting, the real drug or the fake. Patients who thought they were receiving the drug (but were actually taking a placebo) felt relief from their symptoms and experienced immune system elevation. This finding, which has been repeated many times in many different settings throughout medical history, demonstrates how a person's expectations and beliefs affect physiological outcome. If you believe for some reason that you will get better, then you may prove yourself right.

The clinician/client relationship affects treatment outcome as well, because if the patient has a warm, supportive relationship with the clinician, has a positive expectation, and sees the clinician as a knowledgeable partner, the outcome is often positive.[6] If you believe that either the practitioner—or the drug—will help you, then they will. We all need to find caregivers whom we respect and whom we feel can augment our healing process.

How the Immune System Works

Let's look at how the immune system works. White blood cells called lymphocytes are the most important part of the system. Lymphocytes deal with invaders, any dangerous substances that enter into the body. Lymphocytes recognize, destroy, and dispose of foreign invaders such as viruses, bacteria, parasites, and even some cancer cells. One kind of lymphocyte is the macrophage. Its special function is to roam about scouting and searching for things (like virulent flu viruses), recognize them as being foreign bodies, and alert the rest of the immune system that danger is imminent. Macrophages sound the alarm. They engulf the invaders in an effort to destroy them, and alert the rest of the system that something is up.

T cells, which are also important to the immune system, come in many types. Helper T cells are a type of lymphocyte that responds to invaders, like sentries guarding the body. The macrophages alert the Helper T cells to the presence of foreign bodies, germs or bacteria by calling out, "Look! Here comes a flu virus! Do something!" The Helper T's then rouse another kind of lymphocyte, the B cells, who are the decision-makers on this team. The B cells identify the foreign bodies and decide what to do about them. One of their most critical functions is proper identification of the virus or germ. After they have identified the problem, the B cells devise a strategy to drive out the invader (i.e., they develop antibodies that can kill infected cells).

Next in line are the Killer T cells, which actually get rid of the invaders by destroying cancerous and/or virus-infected cells.[7] Killer T's put the plan that the B cells have devised into action. They travel to where the bad cells lurk, destroy them, and signal the rest of the system that everything is okay. Another kind of lymphocyte, called the natural killer cell (scientists call it the NK), can also destroy virus-infected and cancerous cells. All five of these lymphocytes—the macrophage, the Helper T, the Killer T, the B, and the NK—interact with each other in a chain-of-command fashion, and their interconnection is critical. Their teamwork determines the effectiveness of the immune system. Like any organized team, they succeed when pumped up with reinforcements, and they fail on an empty stomach. What drains our immune systems down to an "empty stomach"?—tension, pressure, alcohol, tobacco, lack of exercise, and poor nutrition—to name just a few. What sends in reinforcements?—good diet, exercise, relaxation, and stress reduction techniques which also address our emotional needs.

There are two kinds of immune system malfunctions: immune system disease and auto-immune system disease. Examples of immune system diseases are cancer or AIDS, wherein the system can be so suppressed as to be rendered useless. Auto-immune disease means that the B cells incorrectly identify something as an enemy, when in fact it is a part of the body. Although the "invader" is a part of the body, it is not recognized as such. Because of this mistake, the body attacks a part of itself, and becomes overactive in so doing. Some examples of this are lupus, multiple sclerosis, amyotrophic lateral sclerosis (Lou Gehrig's disease), Hashimotos, fibromyalgia, diabetes, spontaneous infertility, auto-immune AIDS, Addison's disease, and Cushing's syndrome. Addison's disease and Cushing's syndrome both involve the adrenal glands, and these glands can be overstimulated when stress occurs. This is an example of how stress and immunities are interconnected. The similarity between auto-immune and immune disease is this: any time the immune system is not working properly or efficiently, a malfunction of the system transpires. The various aspects of the system must all be working together, coordinated, before an effective response to invasion can happen. If one part malfunctions (as happens when the B cells incorrectly label body tissue as "invader"), the system breaks down. If the macrophages miss an approaching germ, the rest of the team is not roused in time. If the Helper T's are asleep, the B cells aren't notified, and if the B cells miscalculate or don't supply ample tools to the Killer T's, the Killer T's are handicapped.

We know, insofar as we have physiological evidence, that the immune system and the nervous system communicate with each other.[8] This finding suggests to me that what we *think* also influences our cellular functions. Dr. Candace Pert, a molecular biologist formerly at the National Institutes of Health (NIH), and currently a Professor of Molecular and Behavioral Neuroscience at Rutgers University, has been able to show how the neurological system and the immune system send chemical signals to each other, back and forth, in a bidirectional fashion. For Pert, it is not a question of whether or how the mind affects the body, because the mind and the body are *one*—two interconnected parts of the same whole, two inseparable parts of one unified system. The mind and the body cannot help but affect each other.

Pert has studied the way that *peptides* function as *connectors*, or *messengers*, between the mind and the body.

All cells in the body communicate with each other via "messenger" molecules called peptides. (Peptides are composed of amino acids, the building blocks of protein.) In her biological research, Pert has located peptides in the brain as well as in the immune system. Peptides mediate intercellular communication throughout the brain and the body, and some peptides seem to be the biochemical correlates of emotions (when you're grieving, one type of peptide will be in your bloodstream, and when you're ecstatic, a different peptide will be present). Peptide receptors—which peptides seek out because they are a perfect fit—appear on cells all throughout the body, and thus emotions can affect every cell in the body, not just those in our heads. This research tells us that our minds, in a phrase, are in every cell of our bodies. Pert has found peptide receptors on immune cells, and this is why her research suggests there is a relationship between emotions and health. If you've ever been sick over a dying pet or an IRS audit, you already know this.

Pert's findings suggest that any type of bodywork, such as massage, releases peptides into the bloodstream, and this makes intuitive sense to me because I always feel an emotional release after I have a massage. Massage stimulates nerve endings near the skin's surface, so it affects the nervous system, and the nervous system and the immune system are connected by peptide "messengers." Pert's research is particularly interesting when we consider that massage is extolled in Eastern medicine as one of the most ancient methods of healing.[9]

Among Chinese practitioners, massage is a speciality, like pediatrics or radiology. It is not merely a rubdown, but rather a way of addressing imbalance in the body. Chinese massage doctors' hand movements often put pressure on a part of the body quite far away from the symptom, and this has tended to confuse Westerners. How does pressure on the foot affect a pain in the head? Pert's research sheds light on this mystery, and Foot Reflexology, a type of bodywork wherein the feet are massaged, is one example.[10] Nerves run from the brain down through the spinal cord, and then they branch out into the rest of the body, like a river branching into streams. Cells in the nervous system communicate with each other by sending peptide messengers along the neural river and streams. Stimulation of nerve endings in the foot sends messages "upstream" to the brain, and a reflexologist stimulates more than 7000 nerves while working on a person's foot. Pert's research shows how the immune system is affected every time the nervous system is affected, so clearly reflexology could impact upon the immune system.

The part of the nervous system that runs down through the spinal cord is an extension of the brain. Damage to the spinal cord can cause paralysis—loss of movement or feeling in parts of the body that are actually far removed from the spine (e.g., in legs or arms).[11] Without direction from the spinal cord about how and when to act, the muscles do not move. It's as if the neurological river is suddenly dammed up, and little or no information flows through. It seems only logical that if spinal *injury* affects feeling in places far from the spine, spinal *massage* might affect feeling all over the body as well.

Since, as Pert shows, immune cells are linked to nerve cells by peptides, touching the spinal area would inevitably stimulate the immune system. Pert's recent findings, taken together with the historical reputation of massage as a healing technique, might lead us to suspect that the immune system can be enhanced by massage—and maybe that's why it feels so good.

With respect to assessing immune system functioning, blood chemistry and blood counts are the typical methods we use to gauge how the immune system is working, but these are not always the measure of how "well" someone is. I know a woman who has AIDS, and she has no T cells. Nonetheless, she has been alive and well—and functioning—for seven years. How can we explain that? Her white cell count is three thousand, whereas a normal count is five to ten thousand, so you see we cannot always rely on the proverbial "battery of tests." I believe there are other ways to measure how well the immune system is working, and chief among them is simply how well you are functioning, how well you live and resist disease. Laboratory data tell me little about that.

Solomon and Kemeny have studied people like my patient with AIDS for many years. They see people who have been HIV positive for a long time and are still well, with the hope of demystifying exactly what it is that keeps people alive and well. Their research (and that of many other scientists) points to stress—the subject of our next chapter—as a major factor in determining how well we and our immune systems function, and how often we get sick.

—3—

Stress and Its Effects

Your husband offers your spare room to his cousin, a man whose presence you have never enjoyed. Your thalamus—the emotional part of your brain—immediately says, "Get rid of this oaf." Your cortex—the thinking part of your brain—says, "Chill out," or "Be polite. It's only temporary." The more civilized, sophisticated cortex suppresses the thalamus' unbridled urge.

Ah, but hell hath no fury like a thalamus scorned. Rebuffed by the cortex, it turns inward and goes on a silent rampage, inducing your heart to beat rapidly, driving your blood pressure up, and spilling ulcer-causing acids into your stomach. The rebellious thalamus says, in effect, "If you won't do something about this guy, then I will."

Carlton Frederick, PhD, has explained how such conflicts between these two parts of our brain (thalamus and cortex) can decrease the effectiveness of the immune system.[1] The thalamus automatically takes care of many bodily functions for us, so we don't have to remember to breathe every few seconds, make our hearts pump, or constrict our pupils when lights suddenly come on. In addition to performing these basic necessities, the thalamus is also our emotional center, which sometimes means it wants what it wants when it wants it, without consideration for other people, or society as a whole. Like a baby shoving aside precious breakables on her way to a toy, the thalamus' impulse is to grab heedlessly for whatever it desires.

The cortex, on the other hand, is the thinking brain, and it's more socialized. The cortex controls the voluntary muscles, so when the thalamus wants to grab recklessly, the cortex won't allow the hand muscles to reach out. In the case of your cousin-in-law, no matter how much your thalamus wants to tell him to leave, your cortex won't let your mouth say the words. The thalamus is concerned with raw emotion, whereas the cortex is more involved with thoughtfulness. Since the thalamus cannot have its way outright because the cortex denies permission, it turns inward and shakes up things over which it does have control. You find that you cannot sit next to your resident boor without your heart racing (thalamus at work), or your throat tightening (thalamus at work), and one day, without intending to, you "accidentally" spill hot soup on him (thalamus scores small, short-lived victory over cortex). In this manner, whenever the thalamus has a strong urge but cannot act because the cortex won't allow it, the thalamus initiates a process to flood the bloodstream with anxiety-causing chemicals, which eventually hamper the immune system. When our immune systems are depleted and weakened by stress like this, over and over, and then a virus happens by, the immune system is unable to repel it.[2]

I have looked long and hard at the link between stress and the immune system, and a singular truth emerged over and over, wherever I searched. We all have stress; it is a part of life that's not going to go away. At the same time, it is not the amount or severity of stress that matters, but rather the *way we handle our stress* that affects our immune system.

The Stress Response and the Immune System

Certain situations are what we commonly call "distress," whereas other situations are termed "eustress." Eustress is "good" stress, the kind we find exciting or fun. Our perception of the difference between distress and eustress is important. It determines how we handle stress. Hang-gliding and bungee-jumping are eustress for some people, but distress for others. What you might think is distress, I might think is eustress. I like to do lots of things at one time, and this drives some of my friends crazy. They prefer to do one thing at a time, so what is distress for me is eustress for them, and vice versa. Stress, like beauty, is in the eye of the beholder.

If you were to look up suddenly from this book and see a six-hundred pound tiger charging at you with fangs bared, your bloodstream would fill with adrenaline, and you would feel the actual physical result of stress changing your blood chemistry. How does this happen?

There are two subdivisions in the nervous system, the Parasympathetic Nervous Response (PNR) and the Sympathetic Nervous Response (SNR). Our bodies typically operate in the PNR—we work that way under normal conditions and when at rest. The PNR system slows the body down, and aids in digestion, elimination, and relaxation. When stress erupts, the body suddenly jumps into the SNR, also known as the stress response, or the "Fight or Flight" response. (We would instantaneously choose to fight the tiger, or to take flight from him.) The SNR system responds to a stressful situation and speeds up most of the body's responses. During an SNR, our heart rate and blood pressure rise, we feel tense, nauseated, and as if we might faint. The hypothalamus, another part of our brain, releases a chemical called corticotropohormone, and this causes the pituitary to release another chemical called adreno-corticotropohormone, or ACTH. The ACTH then signals the adrenal glands to produce cortisol, beta-endorphins, and epinephrine. Epinephrine reduces interferon, an anti-cancer substance produced by the T cells. Not only is interferon reduced, but in addition we now have all these chemicals surging through our body, and they affect our cytokines. Cytokines are chemical mediators of immune response, involved in notifying the appropriate receptors that it's time to act. Cortisol blocks cytokine production, and this inhibits the white blood cells, since they are dependent upon cytokines to tell them when it's time to go to work. If there is too much distress, the immune system will be suppressed because of the production of all these chemicals. The white blood cells of the immune system (as we discussed in Chapter 2) cannot do their jobs. They are inhibited by lack of cytokines, which were blocked by cortisol, which shot through your system the minute you saw the tiger— or the ornery boss, or the nosy neighbor, or the old lover.

How we handle stress determines how long we remain in the SNR, or how soon we get back to the other side, to a resting state. When the SNR bolts into action, glucose flows abnormally, digestion is inhibited, reproductive growth is decreased, tissue growth and repair are lessened, the cytokines are blocked, and all of this depresses the immune system. The all-important T cells are inhibited by these changes.

The release of hormones during a stress response results in rapid mobilization of energy which flows out in all directions in a massive effort to support the organs and muscles that are fighting to save you from whatever threat has entered the picture.[3] The body stops everything it's doing and runs to the aid of its parts that are spearheading a defense. Normal functions and desires are all set aside while every body part participates in the defense effort. *The immune system is temporarily depressed so that all its energies can be contributed to the problem at hand.* Most of us can withstand this temporary suppression of immune functions, but when long-term, unending stress (e.g., the presence of the unwelcome cousin) results in long-term, unending immune suppression, we cannot fight disease and we can become ill.

The stress response, or SNR, causes changes in the endocrine system (this is why we feel that sudden surge of adrenaline when we see the tiger charging at us); the result is that our behavior and our endocrine system are linked together. Why is this so? The eyes tell the brain that the charging tiger is coming, and the hypothalamus of the brain immediately leaps into action, releasing hormones to activate the parts of the body that need to run, and also to shut down those that are temporarily unnecessary. The hypothalamus, the pituitary gland, and the adrenal glands are all interconnected.[4] When stress arises, the hypothalamus and the adrenal glands work together to release quantities of hormones, such as the aforementioned ACTH, and this release is an endocrine system function.[5] Although the true complexity of the endocrine system is beyond our scope here, this is basically why researchers have found that the release of ACTH and cortisol can be triggered by stress, injury, or illness.[6]

Our bodies respond to stress in two ways: through the nervous system and through the endocrine system. Because they are so closely entwined and interdependent, these two systems are called by one name: the neural-endocrine system. *Nervous system* responses occur between cells via chemical transmitters, while *endocrine* responses involve the hormones just mentioned. The hypothalamic-pituitary-adrenal connection—or as scientists call it, the hypothalamic-pituitary axis—is in fact a *convergence* of neural and hormonal adaptive mechanisms to help the body to manage or adjust to stressors. So there is no way the mind and the body could react separately to stress; they are literally tied together.

(The neurons in the hypothalamus have many connections with the central nervous system, and the peptides as discussed in Chapter 2 function along these connections.)

Events that cause stress, for us and for our neural-endocrine systems, can originate either outside the body (e.g., external events) or inside the body (e.g., sugar overload); diabetes is one example of this.

Too much sugar is as fatally stressful to a diabetic as the charging tiger, even though the sugar is inside the body and the tiger is outside. For a diabetic, sugar is a stressor. Although less fatal for many, to some degree sugar is a stressor for all of us. Sugar intake stimulates the pancreas to secrete insulin, and the blood sugar drops. This causes the liver to produce glycogen (stored sugar), which then stimulates the adrenal glands, so the whole hypothalamic-pituitary-adrenal (or neural-endocrine) system becomes involved. It follows that too much sugar in the blood on a constant basis can eventually lead to overworking the adrenal glands, which eventually affects the whole system.[7] Continued stress, whether it comes from inside or out, forces the pancreas and the rest of the neural-endocrine system into hyperactivity, and our bodies are not designed to deal with constant stress.[8]

What this all means is that stress does play a role in altering blood sugar levels. Physicians who treat stockbrokers have noted that they do not need to read newspapers to find out what's happening on Wall Street; they can tell by the amount of sugar excreted by diabetic brokers (a sort of Mind-Body-Market Indicator). Aerial combat has been observed to cause transient diabetes in army pilots.[9] Again, these are examples of the interconnections between the thalamic brain, the pituitary gland, the adrenal gland, and the pancreas. Our neural-endocrine systems are designed to manage *sudden* deviations in blood sugar levels—indeed, sudden surprise is exactly what elicits an SNR—but not *continual* deviations, as diabetes and unwelcome cousins both prove.[10] Again, one of the problems with *continual* stress, whether it comes from inside or outside the body, is that the immune system becomes depressed.

Can you think of anything that might spur on a stress response? How about children, husbands, lovers, ex-husbands, finances, jobs, lack of jobs, illnesses, lack of love, doing too much, trauma, assault, abuse, reading the newspapers, or watching TV? Which foods trigger the (internal) stress response?—sugar, caffeine, dairy products, and alcohol. The three worst offenders are sugar, caffeine, and alcohol. If you are feeling anxious a great deal of the time, you may be creating the SNR by drinking caffeine or sugar, both of which stimulate the adrenals. The combination of sugar and caffeine together, as found in colas and coffee with sugar, is particularly problematic, for while caffeine adversely affects the adrenals, sugar is simultaneously causing overactivity in the pancreas.[11] There are compelling reasons to examine exactly what we put into our bodies. Can you identify what is causing a stress response? Is it food? A relationship? Your job?

Handling Stress Effectively

I spoke to a breast cancer survivor who told me the hardest part was worrying that she might have cancer when she found a lump. But once she found out it was cancerous, she knew just what to do, and she busied herself getting well. She said, "We women can handle these things really well." That's not to say that men cannot, but in this instance, her belief that she "could handle it" enabled her to do just that. This is a fundamental example of the Mind/Body Connection, and of handling stress effectively.

We have the mechanisms and the support systems we need to deal with stress intelligently, but often, we think we don't. We think that we are all alone. We become overwhelmed by our troubles and no longer believe we know what to do, yet we have tools we can use to deal with stress, elevate the immune system response, and thereby improve our overall level of wellness. It's as if we have the equipment, but we are reluctant to actually take it out of the toolbox. A hammer does not get up and pound a nail by itself. We need to take advantage of the resources within and around us.

Bodywork can be an effective stress reduction technique. This means massage or any procedure wherein patients are touched by the health professional. Massage is an ancient form of healing, and now we know that it actually releases peptides into the blood and muscles and thereby elevates the immune response. New York University Professor of Nursing, Dolores Krieger, has done numerous studies on therapeutic touch, and she finds that touch does help to heal.[12] She found that patients who are touched more frequently in the hospital go home sooner. Premature babies who are touched frequently, in their incubators, also gain weight faster. It seems we have become so isolated, so busy, and so fearful of inappropriate touches, that we don't touch each other at all any more. Krieger developed her theory of therapeutic touch as an approach to healing the whole person after observing a healer, Oskar Estebany, relieve people's pain by moving his hands over them. She became convinced that this skill could be learned and since the 1970s has taught many courses in therapeutic touch. Taking her lead, several universities and continuing education programs offer formal instruction in therapeutic touch to practitioners from many different fields.

In Krieger's courses, the person providing touch learns to "center themselves" and to focus their healing energies into the process to be conducted. The healer places his or her hands over the patient, four to six inches above the patient's body, and attempts to visualize a field of positive, healing energy. Krieger observed that, at the very least, the process results in relaxation for people suffering from severe pain, fever, inflammation, or psychosomatic symptoms. Dr. Janet Quinn of the University of Colorado conducted a study on the effects of therapeutic touch in 1985, and the healers who were able to center themselves, in her study, reported they felt energy pass between themselves and the patients. Patients reported a noticeable drop in anxiety levels.[13]

Acupuncture is another tool we can use to defuse stress. It involves touching in addition to the use of very thin needles (no thicker than a strand of hair). The goal is to elevate the immune response by creating balance in the body's energy system.[14] Yoga can also be used to regain a sense of balance.[15]

There are different types of massage and touch therapies. Feldenkreis, Rolfing, Reiki, auric-balancing, and Rosen are just a few. Rosen was developed specifically to release old patterns and beliefs through the movement of various muscle groups. Reiki is a type of energy treatment which resembles therapeutic touch because it involves healing with hands. The practitioner places her hands around the client's energy field in order to allow energy to pass from the universe through her to the client. I have felt both physical and emotional releases following Reiki treatments many times. For patients who do not understand Reiki, it might be uncomfortable or even difficult to imagine. But for many people, including myself, Reiki feels tremendously healing.

Meditation, like the various types of massage, has been considered effective, for thousands of years in some cultures, because it reduces the stress response. Sitting quietly and breathing slowly can shift the body away from the SNR and back into the PNR. Meditation means not having a crowd of stress-inducing chemicals bubbling around in the bloodstream and stirring up all manner of trouble. By meditating regularly, you can fairly often keep your body in a state of quiet and rest with all systems operating at normal speed. How important this can be in terms of illness! When you are under a lot of stress, even when the stress is the presence of illness itself, meditation will allow fewer of those chemicals from the adrenal glands to make their merry way through your bloodstream.

Jon Kabat Zinn operates what he calls a "pain clinic" at the University of Massachusetts.[16] Patients are referred to this clinic by their doctors. Zinn teaches patients meditation and yoga, and this often diminishes their pain. These are people who have lived with excruciating pain, sometimes for years, and who have sought every type of relief known to medical science with no success. Zinn's patients report that they can make decisions better after meditating, because there is not so much angst and anxiety clouding their vision.

The experience of illness is daunting. You can get so anxious about your pain that you cannot "think straight." When this occurs, it helps to slow down and take deep breaths. *Slow breathing is a bridge between the mind and the body.* Slow breathing has also been shown to force the release of toxins from the body.[17] This good riddance may also elevate the immune response.

The effects of hypnosis have been analyzed with melanoma patients as subjects.[18] Those patients who underwent hypnosis had a reduced rate of recurrence, suggesting that this is another technique which heals by quieting us down and providing respite from the pace of our frantic lives. A further advantage is that hypnosis can help us to recall old traumas that we might be suppressing, or holding onto inside our bodies, allowing us then to seek release from them, because old traumas can literally make us sick. They are sometimes involved in the development of auto-immune disease, which occurs, as we mentioned in Chapter 2, when our immune system mistakenly attacks a part of our own body.

Chronic Fatigue Syndrome (CFS) is one type of auto-immune disease. I saw a patient who was overwhelmed and overcommitted, and was suffering from CFS. She had two children and was working full time to support the whole family. I questioned her about her childhood, and discovered that her life had been riddled with abuse and trauma. I asked if she had ever thought about the impact of her childhood issues on her current problems, but she had not. My opinion with regard to her CFS, an auto-immune disease, was that her body was eating itself up as a result of psychological issues she had harbored and held onto for so long, and the situation was aggravated by her current state of exhaustion. I suggested counseling as the first step toward healing what had by this point become a physical illness. The Mind-Body Connection is an initial aspect that needs to be addressed at the onset of what seem to be only bodily symptoms.

As we move through life, we find that aging can be stressful because it brings considerable changes in our abilities and our looks. Although we usually relate age with infirmity, this is, in fact, as much a cultural belief as it is an objective observation. But aging does not have to involve infirmity. As we study elderly people who are living in good health, for instance, we find, as Deepak Chopra has observed, that autonomy is very important. Being able to make their own decisions and live their own lives is a factor common to people who live into their late 80s and 90s (see Chapter 2). Such elderly people believe in being fighters, being optimistic, getting information, processing it individually, and making personal choices. Solomon, as mentioned earlier, has also studied older populations and found that people who have goals live longer and healthier lives.

Those of us who genuinely try to "feel our feelings" and get honest with ourselves about our emotions can help our immune system to function by doing so. You cannot parrot platitudes such as "I have a positive attitude," while inside you're furious with someone, or about something. *The mouth cannot trick the mind, or the body, with socially acceptable utterances.* I cannot emphasize enough how essential it is to be honest with yourself about what is going on in your heart of hearts. If you are angry, or sad, or happy, you cannot fool your body about that fact. If the mind and body are always connected, and are one and the same, how could it be any different? Whatever is going on in the mind needs to be expressed. If it does not find expression through the mouth, then it will surely emerge as an ulcer, rash, or some other symptom.

This does not mean you go out and shoot everybody in town if you're angry. It means that you say, if only to yourself, "I'm angry. I am truly angry," instead of "Well, it doesn't really bother me that she got the promotion instead of me, or that my husband came home late, or, or, or . . ." We need to identify anger as a legitimate emotion, and to deal with it in an appropriate manner without hurting somebody else. This is true for current anger as well as for anger that may be left over from the distant past. Some HIV positive people I know, and many with CFS, seek out treatments such as Primal Scream Therapy, for one, which forces feelings to burst out. They attempt to work with very old traumas that they may not be fond of. It is important to pull for whatever is down there in the depth of your soul that has not been addressed. We cannot relax in our current life, no matter how much meditation or slow breathing we do, if we are secretly fuming about something that hurt us twenty years ago. We have all had traumas, we have all had issues, and it is *healthful* to try to see what needs to be healed, no matter how uncomfortable it is to think about.

As important as facing our psychological issues is to our health, we must also remember that it is equally important to get on with our lives and try to have fun. Research has shown again and again that humor improves immune system functions.[19] Every time you laugh, endorphins are released, and this has a positive impact on health. Endorphins are brain chemicals that help us in many ways.[20] Let's think about some things that might elevate the immune system in this regard. There's dancing, exercise, walking, hugging, seeing a friend, kissing, singing, praying, having capacity for joy, creative work, and healthy relationships.

Speaking of relationships, they are probably the biggest stressor for most people, because they are the thing we worry about most. Being socially involved and communally connected with others improves our immune responses, so it is worthwhile to make an effort not to sit home alone and be despondent. Connecting with other people does help, because any activity that helps our mind also simultaneously helps our body. More and more medical evidence suggests that this is a law of nature.[21]

And while we are on the subject of being with other people, we should note that support groups can ease the travails of life in a variety of situations. Support groups basically consist of people with similar problems coming together and utilizing the "Talking Cure." Getting things "off your chest," as the old saying goes, is healing. (There's a reason why these things are *old* sayings; they have worked for a *long* time.) For example, studies have suggested that women with breast cancer who attend support groups tend to live longer and to have more meaningful lives than those women who do not join groups.[22] At the Commonweal Cancer Help Program, in Bolinas, California, people with life-threatening diseases come and live together for a full week, form friendships, and speak with each other at length about their lives and fears. The Program is not a type of therapy, but is rather more educational. To be eligible to attend, patients must be under the care of an oncologist or other qualified physician. Many are undergoing cancer treatment and some have been told there's nothing more that medicine can do for them. They go to Commonweal to determine *what they can do for themselves* at this difficult point in their lives.[23] Patients I have spoken with claim they left Commonweal feeling that the week had changed their lives in terms of quality of relationships. They were able to take what they had learned home to their families and friends, and thus their relationships outside the group were positively affected. They had learned how to get honest.

It's worthwhile noting that having pets can elevate the immune response, too, because animals can be calming and nurturing, and as such they provide comfort to someone suffering stress, illness, or both. They give unconditional love and they usually don't argue back. Gardening is another activity that is relaxing and curative. Bubble baths, too, serve the same purpose, and you undoubtedly can think of a few other stress reduction techniques that work for *you* personally.

Getting Information about Illness as a Way to Decrease Stress

It is increasingly clear that we need to take responsibility for our own health care, and that we don't leave all decision making to health care professionals (including myself). It's not the physician's life, or the nurse's body, or the X-ray technician's marriage that is at stake, it's yours. Medical practitioners don't always understand what is happening with you specifically. Remember: you are a whole person with a life, relationships, spiritual beliefs, and feelings, and therefore you should be the one to look at what options are available for you, and then make your own decisions.

A man I knew went to a physician and was told he was HIV positive. The doctor said, "We're going to use AZT treatments, and this is the plan I have for you." The patient said, "No, I don't think so. I prefer a holistic approach." The doctor said, "You're crazy, and you're going to die." So the patient got up out of the chair, and said, "Thank you very much, but you're no longer my doctor." He left the office; he's been HIV positive for six years, and he's doing well. He's not sick, he has no symptoms or physical problems. He has adopted a holistic philosophy about his condition, and he has made choices that he felt were right for him. He did not do what a doctor felt was right, but what *he* felt was right. This brings me to my next point: you need to decide for yourself what it is that works for you.

When you enter a health care setting, you are usually given just one choice. The doctor might say, "You need to have surgery." This conventional approach is important in the treatment of many illnesses, and should not be ignored. However, you also need to consider what I call the "other side" of illness, and to decide what else you might want to do in addition to the more traditional treatments such as surgery, chemotherapy, or radiation. The research repeatedly shows that people with *choices*, people who could make choices for themselves, rather than being told what to do by a practitioner, win more battles in the war against disease.[24] The goal of my practice is to help people sort out their alternatives and choices, and to assist them in making decisions about holistic and/or conventional therapies.

Trusting a care-giver is a crucial issue. When patients perceive their care-givers as authority figures who know what they are talking about, and when the authority says, "This is what works, and this is what we have seen in the research," patients respond trustingly to that authority. This confirms that it is essential to find practitioners with whom you feel comfortable. It is your right as a patient! If you do not feel comfortable, stress is created in your body, and this leads right back to a fight between the nervous system and the immune system. We can probably all recall how it feels to be in the presence of a practitioner we do not respect, who is telling us things we do not agree with. If you do not feel a sense of teamwork between you and your practitioner, it would be better to change to another practitioner you do trust.

Recently, I saw a young girl as a patient who had an unusually large cyst on her ovary. A sonogram indicated that it might be malignant. She told me she did not want to have it surgically removed, although that is the typical procedure in cases with a suggestive sonogram. Together, we examined a range of possibilities. I suggested to her that she keep getting opinions until she found a practitioner she really trusted. She needed to be at ease with the information she was getting, and only then could she proceed with treatment. She called some time later and reported that, because of our discussions, she had finally found someone who did eventually perform surgery. She had to travel quite a distance in her quest. The cyst was not a tumor, but rather endometriosis. She was pleased with the outcome, and very glad that she had taken the extra time to look around and find someone with whom she felt comfortable. We should not underestimate this factor, because it is so relevant to healing.

Health care professionals have different philosophies about what works and what does not work. I might say to a patient, "Have you considered acupuncture?" If the patient is terrified of needles, the very idea would be stressful. Acupressure, which is done without needles, might work better. After years of working as a nurse and a nurse practitioner, I have learned to listen to patients' needs and feelings about things, and I have come to understand that *listening is essential to curing.*

Carl Simonton is a scientist who studies the link between what he calls "visualizations" and illness.[25] His patients are instructed to visualize their immune systems, and to visualize the good cells eating up the bad cells. One patient claimed that, since he was a pacifist, he "could not imagine anything eating up anything else. So I'm going to invite the bad cells to politely leave my body." However we deal with this issue, we do need to take the information that we receive and decide what works best for us specifically, as unique individuals. Of course, what works for one person does not necessarily work for another. Our bodies will tell us what works, although they may have to tell us over and over and over before we listen.

I provide my patients with as much information as possible to help them make choices. My advice is, "This is like a deck of cards. I hand you all the possible cards, and you pick the winning hand for you." The winning hand is different for each of us, because we have different lives, different health histories, and different belief systems. We need to get to the truth of what is right for us, not what is right for someone else, or a dozen "someone elses." In this respect, each woman must find her own safe place for healing.

Depending on the situation, I sometimes suggest to a patient that she look into the use of herbal or homeopathic remedies. Homeopathy is the use of naturally occurring herbs or plants to treat illness.[26] Generally these herbs and/or plant leaves are encapsulated into pills, or tea bags, and sold in health food stores. Many people have found relief from skin rashes, infections, bites, gastritis, and other common physical and stress-related disorders by using homeopathic remedies. Practitioners of herbal or homeopathic medicine are often listed in holistic health care guides or in telephone directories. Although there are books published on homeopathy, I recommend supervised use, since it is a complicated science.

I might also just as readily encourage a patient to consult a surgeon for more conventional treatment. The point is this: every illness is different, every person is different, and everyone's stress is different. We need to open our minds to the notion of considering every possible option. When we are sick, why shouldn't we avail ourselves of every solution known to medicine, whether it be a laser treatment patented yesterday, or an herb recipe that's worked for five thousand years? Often a combination of both conventional and non-conventional treatments leads to a cure.

You may already have some intuitive feelings about stress and illness. You may have felt that you really know what made you sick. Nonetheless, we are all so accustomed to accepting a technical explanation, that we may too easily accept it, and slide again into old habits. Now you can say, "See, I was right.

The scientific research says so." The research just proves what we already know, that the mind and body are one, and what you think and what you say and how you live does affect how long you will live and what quality of life you will have. The words we use, the words we put forth, do affect us. Negative words and words of doubt, such as "I don't think I can," may suppress our spontaneity and with it our immune system as well. The immune system is like an athletic team. If you concentrate on charging up its enthusiasm, what do you think will happen?

Listening to Your Body

The Killer T cells in our system need to be mobilized. The way to do that is to take the steps we have mentioned, to really get in there and win health back. Since we are all going to die, the quality of life we have while we are alive is all that matters. At the same time, I believe that we all know how to improve our quality of life, but we rarely do because we think we don't. I am constantly surprised by the number of women who come to me on a regular basis thinking they don't know what is hurting them. I say to them, "You do know. Tell me what you think is going on. Listen to your body and it will tell you what is out of balance."

Over the years, several tests have been developed to measure illness indicators in people who are under stress.[27] They measure the connection between illness and factors like death, divorce, marriage, or bankruptcy. The higher the score, the greater the risk that illness may develop. For its part, the medical community has studied the controversial idea of using these measurements to determine if there is a relationship between stress and disease. I have worked in health care for thirty years and for me there is no question about it. There is an enduring relationship. Stress causes biochemical reactions to occur in the body, and eventually these wear the body out, and then illness develops.

We are not going to eliminate stress, so what are we going to do? If we don't address the stress somehow, it will stay in the body. The mind and the body are one, and this is why your cells will know when you are overstressed. We cannot hide it from them, although we surely try. We need to learn to manage our stress, which means getting it out of our bodies, since it is not going to disappear by itself. We lead complicated, fast-paced lives thanks to computers, car phones, FAX machines, and all manner of media intrusion. It just may be that our nervous systems were not necessarily designed to move so quickly. All this hyperactivity may overtax the immune system and thus set us up for disease, unless we slow down or make anti-stress techniques a priority in our lives. What you do or don't do about this can and does make a difference.

—4—

Codependency
and Illness

Sunlight sparkled everywhere, sprinkling shades of tangerine, lemon, and violet over the flowers outside, but I sat indoors staring at the mirror, numb, as if it were a rainy midnight at the end of the world. My reflection broadcast a basal cell carcinoma right on my face. I saw it there, I knew it was there, I knew exactly what it was; I had been seeing it there for six months, I knew I had been seeing it there for six months, and I knew I had been ignoring it or pretending not to see what I saw. If a patient of mine took care of herself this way, I would tell her to run, not walk, to therapy.

I had been in a love affair with a man who made me many promises about "our future together." He told me he would "be there" for me, but he was never "there," or anywhere, for me. I believed him even though the things he promised never came to be. The difference between his promises and reality grew wider and wider until it was like the Grand Canyon. I was totally committed to him and focused on him and his needs. I felt obsessed and addicted and so "in love" with the fantasy of our being together. Now that it was over, I saw how much I had ignored my own needs—to the point of not getting medical attention for a potentially malignant growth. In retrospect, too, I now believe the suppressed anger and hurt feelings lowered my interferon level, depleting my immune system, and allowed the carcinoma to advance untempered. (As Joan Borysenko's research has shown, when interferon levels are low, the immune system cannot prevent the growth of cancer cells to the degree that it normally does.[1]) I had tried to excuse myself over the issue of cost. I felt I could not afford to have the carcinoma removed; I would see to it when I had the money. Then I remembered I had taken a ski trip, and the cost of the airfare would have paid for the surgery. Not only that, I also had insurance to cover costs. How could I afford a vacation but not medical necessities? Only upside down priorities and denial of my feelings made that kind of financial decision possible. A few weeks later, I began to realize that my confusion wasn't over money, but about something else. I finally sought out a plastic surgeon who is a friend and colleague.[2] After injecting a local anesthetic, he surgically removed a wide piece of skin that included the cancerous lesion and surrounding tissue. Then I had to wait for an hour to hear the pathology report. When it finally came back, we found out it was only a low-grade basal cell carcinoma; however, it had been inadequately excised. The surgeon had to remove more tissue and then I had to wait another hour for the second report. Finally, good news arrived. All the malignant cells had been removed. Fortunately, my surgeon was kind and supportive throughout this anxiety-producing experience. I seem to be completely cured and have only a minimal scar, thanks to his expertise. It was a financially and emotionally expensive lesson—one I hope not to repeat. It was a wake-up call about my patterns of codependency.

I started thinking while under the surgeon's knife, and I knew that I had let the cancer grow for so long because I could not face it or myself. I ignored my own needs and allowed stress to drive down my immunities. I call this codependency.

What Exactly Is It?

Codependency means caring for others, while we ignore our own needs and symptoms, to the point of becoming ill.[3] This is

a particularly insidious situation for women who have been so-
cietally oriented toward codependency, as if it were positive
and healthy. Remember "Miss Congeniality"? (As if we could
forget.) Addressing codependency as it affects health means
taking responsibility for our own behavior, for setting our own
limits and boundaries.

When we become ill, we usually avail ourselves of the technical wonders of conventional medicine. It seems miraculous
that we can be at death's door one day, and twenty-four hours
later on the road to recovery, all because of rubbing in some
pharmaceutical liniment, or submitting to minor surgery. The
dazzling glare of the miracle blinds us to the way in which
codependency makes us so sick that only a miracle will save us.
*My concern about codependency and illness is that the connec-
tion between them is too frequently an unrecognized phenome-
non in conventional medical practices.*

When patients recount a variety of physical complaints, the
first thing I do is to ask them what is going on in their lives and
relationships for them to feel so bad. I then outline the possibility of a connection between what is going on in their lives
and relationships and their physical complaints—their somatic
complaints, that is. ("Somatic" means physical, or bodily. The
more commonly heard term "psychosomatic" means the inter-
action of mental and bodily phenomena—as in "psychosomatic
ulcers"—and does not mean it is all in one's head.) People are
always amazed to hear this, as if the mind and body were not
connected. In conventional medical practices, few practitioners question patients about what is going on in their lives and
whether it might be related to their symptoms. A full gambit of
costly medical tests is performed, and often there is nothing

wrong, according to the laboratory data. Then both patient and practitioner grow puzzled. Our own bodies tell us long before the lab tests that something is wrong, but we are often too out of touch with our bodies, and/or so focused on everyone else, that we ignore the warning signals.

In cases where something is found to be wrong, the tumor is removed, or the lumpectomy is done, or radiation and chemotherapy are administered, and *still* no one asks the patient how she's feeling. How does she behave? What does she think? Does she have a primary relationship? What is going on in that relationship? Does she have children? Is she codependent in her relationships, and how does that affect her health? What are her feelings and does she have a mechanism to deal with them?

Codependent Patterns of Living

In her writing, Louise Hay has often pointed out that if you don't address the underlying problem, you may create another illness.[4] I have found this to be true both personally and with women I see in my practice. I believe it is critical to discuss with women their possible patterns of codependency, and to refer them to counselors who can explore the potentially physical impact of these issues. My observation over eleven years of holistic women's health care practice is that codependency means being overly concerned with others' lives and consequently ignoring immediate, personal needs. If we concentrate on someone else's problems, that's a convenient way to avoid looking at our own problems, and this can make us sick. If we are codependent, we cannot adequately resolve our own vexa-tions. Indeed, we are usually not even aware of our own stress because we pour our energies into someone else's stress, or their job, or their sickness, or their love life. Managing our own stress requires taking time out to look at our own lives instead of zealous devotion someone else's.

In her book, *A Different Voice*, author Carol Gilligan sug-gests that women derive much of their identity from relation-ships.[5] I have observed when relationships are strained that women may experience physical symptoms and stress responses. While a certain number of readers will predictably dismiss this notion as hocus-pocus, I see examples of it every day. Many women come to me with vaginitis, fibroids, endometriosis, or breast masses, and these symptoms are frequently accompanied by relationship issues. Sometimes women who are unhappy in their primary relationships don't know what to do. They don't want to leave their partners, and they would like to talk about their feelings, but they don't know how, or their partners are un-interested or unresponsive. I've seen women like this develop chronic vaginitis, which I treat repeatedly. I talk to them about conventional drugs and holistic prevention, but the core of the problem may be quite different, and may require identifying what they are not dealing with in their lives, and what they may be submerging into their gynecological organs. What does re-current vaginitis tell us? It's possible that we're not eating well because we're too busy to take care of ourselves. It's also possi-ble we are in an unsatisfying, uncomfortable, or abusive relation-ship, and we are unable to discuss our feelings. We may have work that we absolutely hate and don't know how to get out of, or we may not know how to quit a job and start a new career. When

enduring the effects of consistent, ever increasing, stress, inno-
cent cells may eventually cave in.

A therapist taught me how many women carry repressed
rage around when he asked me if I could verbalize my anger.
He said he had seen many women with repressed rage who
could not express it after being taught to be "nice" girls.
Women are often taught not to speak up, not to be angry, and to
"make everything nice." When he asked me to identify and express my rage and anger, I was mystified. Anger? What does
that mean? How do I get at it? And *what will happen to my relationships, or to me, if I express it?* Was I different from any
other woman? I doubted it. But as I calmed down, I felt it, an
unmistakable burning from somewhere deep within me. Giving voice to my feelings also clarified them and how I could resolve them.

The symptoms derived from repressed anger are diverse. In
my patients as in myself, I have long noticed how repressed
anger can lead to depression and physical disease. Dis-ease literally means "without ease" or "lack of ease." The generally ac-
cepted role that women play in society—as caretakers or
nurturers—can be wonderfully rewarding if not taken to the ex-
treme. *But when a woman nurtures (or interferes) to the point
of not nurturing herself, it takes a toll on her body.*

There is reason for this, too, and it is borne out time and
again: Women usually do not speak up about what is going on
inside them. Perhaps the risk is too great—to herself, her self-
image, to others? Anger can seem terrible when we do not give
it voice. In the same sense, when we cannot vent our feelings,
we put them into our bodies. As Melanie Beattie argued in her
book, *Codependent No More,* the core of this issue also involves

focusing outward to care for and about others instead of inward to care for and about ourselves.[6] If we don't speak up about our anger, our sadness, our frustration, our needs, where does all that energy go? Where do these feelings go? They go into our bodies, as we discussed in Chapter 2. We should remember that codependency works best in silence and requires that we not speak up. Congeniality can sometimes be quite brutal at heart.

In a study of adolescent girls' responses to questions about feelings, Gilligan found that the girls initially would not answer forthrightly. Regardless of what she asked, they responded with some version of "I don't know." After repeated attempts, Gilligan managed to build some sense of trust between herself and the girls, and they began to speak up. They did in fact know everything that was happening to them, but they were afraid to verbalize for fear of losing their boyfriends, their peers, or of angering their parents. So they pretended not to know. Gilligan's contention, that women are taught from their earliest years not to know, for fear of losing relationships, and men are taught to suppress or submerge what they know, is clear enough. But knowing and doing are too different too much of the time. We need to stop pretending not to know what is going on, and stop suppressing feelings when we do know. If women could stop pretending not to know and speak up, as my experience as a nurse tells me, they may have fewer physical complaints.

Awareness and the Modern Medical Diagnosis

Experience has led me to believe that women sometimes put issues of the heart into their pelvis, and ovarian cysts are one example. A common condition for many women, ovarian cysts are generally benign and require minimal treatment. Symptoms include pelvic pain, irregular menses, and leg pain. The typical care is to observe the cyst in a biannual exam, order a sonogram to determine its size and any unusual aspects, and then to monitor its growth in subsequent exams. Birth control pills have been successfully used to lessen the size of cysts. Acupuncture and herbs have also been effective. Western medicine, though, has not been able to determine what causes ovarian cysts. When a woman comes to see me with a cyst, I always ask her to tell me about her relationships—what is going on in them and how she feels about them. I encourage women especially to evaluate their feelings about love relationships. Are they holding on to any anger or sadness which needs to be expressed? Very often, I find that to be the case.

Ovarian cysts often bring to the surface women's great fear of ovarian cancer, particularly since the death of celebrity Gilda Radner garnered so much publicity about it. I explain to patients that ovarian cancer is an extremely rare disease, and difficult to diagnose early. Presently, there are only two tests which can lead to early diagnosis: the CA 125 blood test and a sonogram. The symptoms of ovarian cancer are abdominal bloating, back pain, and unusual bleeding, although a woman can have all these symptoms and not have ovarian cancer. If a woman is suspicious, she should be offered both these tests and then make her own decision based on the costs and her intuition. Christiane Northrup refers to ovarian cancer as the Golden Handcuff Syndrome, since it is often linked to women who stay married to wealthy men for financial reasons, despite enormous unhappiness—another codependency related illness.[7]

Another common gynecological complaint that often seems linked to codependent stress is urinary tract infections (UTIs). The symptoms are pain with urination, frequent urination, blood in the urine, pain with intercourse, itching, and fever. The conventional treatment is 3 to 7 days on antibiotics. Holistic treatment makes use of the herbs Golden Seal, Uva Ursi, and marshmallow root 3 times daily for 3 to 7 days. Causative factors include not drinking enough liquids leading to infrequent urination, as well as sex, sugar, alcohol, stress, and the tendency for women to ignore their bodies when they are too busy. One patient of mine suffered recurrent UTIs until, during our discussions together about her relationship, she realized that she was literally "pissed off" at her boyfriend and her bladder was letting her know it.

Another patient suffered from undiagnosed chronic pelvic pain. I talked to her about whether or not she had been sexually abused. Sometimes women know they have been abused, other times they don't know they've been abused, and other times they may have imagined their abuse. Deepak Chopra and Christiane Northrup have both proposed that our cells store the memory of everything that has ever happened to them.[8] Eventually, through some physical symptom, the body may express a prior trauma which has not been acknowledged. I have seen women who have suppressed or not talked about sexual trauma, and then for some reason began to remember the event. They start to "know" themselves, without a doctor telling them, that pelvic pain or other chronic gynecological conditions are psychogenic (meaning they start in the mind). They gradually come to feel they need to see a psychological counselor (not a pharmaceutical fix) to help heal what has, over time, become a physical manifestation.

Because of the mind's powerful ability to imagine, deny, or suppress sexual abuse, many women are not aware that anything happened to them as children. They come to me with complaints of pelvic pain which I am unable to diagnose. Their physical tests come back negative from the laboratory. The exam proves they have pain but we cannot find a reason. Often I treat them with a round of antibiotics and they get better for a while, but eventually the pain returns. The body is the storehouse for those essential wounds the mind (and the mouth) cannot express.

Speaking of things the mouth would rather not discuss brings me to the subject of fibroids and divorce.

I have come to believe that uterine fibroids can be the culmination of years of being plugged into a codependent relationship, where women experience blocked creativity and blocked feelings because they are so locked into caring for or overprotecting their partners. I see a growing number of women with fibroids of the uterus, and I see a pattern of fibroids linked with divorce. Fibroids are benign masses which enlarge the uterus, tend to increase periods, cause pelvic pain, and make it difficult to pass urine or move the bowels. Often these fibroids are nothing to worry about, technically speaking, but they cause extraordinary practical problems. Fibroids sometimes appear to accompany repressed anger. Northrup suggests they are related to dead-end jobs or relationships. When I talk to these women about their relationships, I frequently discover they are having romantic troubles, getting divorced, or dislike their work. They are experiencing sadness, anger, and feelings they never acknowledge. I encourage them to look at holistic medicine, to let their bodies teach them what they need to know.

Herbal practitioners, also called naturopaths, have had some success treating fibroids with herbs, accompanied by counseling to release anger. Acupuncture can relieve fibroids. I find that as women start to deal with these issues, to thoughtfully and persistently move these feelings out of the body, the fibroids shrink. Despite this, holistic treatments are not generally addressed in conventional gynecology. My experience is that holistic approaches to treating fibroids can be significantly effective. A woman has to be motivated and prepared to do a great deal of work emotionally, as well as committed to taking herbs and possibly acupuncture. These can be colossal steps for some of us.

Conventional scientific wisdom tends to correlate fibroids with age. Thus, scientists might counter psychogenic explanations with the fact that 20% to 50% of all women eventually develop fibroids anyway, even if they do *not* get divorced.[9] However, I have seen too many fibroids follow divorce to continue to believe that it's just "coincidence." That would be like looking down at my five fingers and saying, "No, I have only four."

Endometriosis is overgrowth of the uterine lining; eventually, the enlarged lining moves outside of the uterus. Endometriosis can be caused by excessive production of estrogen from animal fats, stress, or other unknown factors. Estrogen overproduction stimulates proliferation (growth and thickening) of the lining—the endometrium—and this overgrowth migrates outside the uterus to other parts of the abdomen. The overgrowth and movement causes heavy periods, brownish irregular spotting, pelvic and menstrual pain, as well as pain during intercourse. Like fibroids, it often seems to be related to codependent relationships, and may be considered a stress-related illness in women, since we submerge many of our relationship feelings into our pelvic organs. In ancient medical practices that divide the body into different areas called "chakras," the pelvic chakra is the second chakra, which is all about relationships.[10] It makes sense to me that we as women would push unexpressed feelings about affairs of the heart into what I consider the other heart of women, their gynecological organs. When we *listen* to our bodies, we begin to recognize that illness may not be a random event. Illness is a teacher, guiding us toward needed changes. Perhaps we need to say "no" to others and to their endless demands, to set limits in our relationships, and set boundaries on our volunteer time. Illness is a lifeboat sent out to save us. We don't have to get aboard. We can choose to ignore it, continuing to thrash about in the sea of secret emotions and temporary cures, and hope we don't drown.

For many years now, physiological and medical researchers have observed the relationship between stressful events and the progression of cancer in animal subjects as well as in humans.[11] In her books *Codependent No More* and *Beyond Codependency,* Melanie Beattie describes what may be a link between codependency and cancer. Long ago I noticed that many cancer patients had suffered major losses, such as the loss of a loved one. In the context of breast cancer especially, I saw connections to the death of a spouse, or to a traumatic love relationship with a parent or lover. I have long harbored a suspicion that increasing rates of breast cancer may somehow be related to some women's inability to take care of themselves, and to their need to focus outward toward the care of someone else. This creates an imbalance between giving and receiving. What happens when that other someone dies? What do they focus on then? There are many causes of breast cancer and all disease is multifactorial. I do not suggest that an imbalance between giving and receiving is the only cause. Nevertheless, there is a commonality here that may reveal much about the body, disease, and culture.

Breasts, I believe, are about relationships and nurturing for women. Christiane Northrup cites the intriguing case of a woman in her 60s with nipple discharge. The woman's daughter had recently moved away from home. Northrup analyzed the discharge, which turned out to be breast milk. The nurturing of her daughter, and the inevitable empty nest, had created stress in the woman's body. As a mother, she was accustomed to worrying about her daughter's care and welfare. She was unable to talk about her sense of loss, and she put it into her body.[12]

I've seen quite a few women with unusual bleeding of the uterus and I always ask them about their relationships, because the ancient Chinese medical belief is that unusual bleeding is about an affair of the heart.[14] So many women will say to me, "I can't believe you asked me that, because I just broke up with my lover," or "My father just died." I believe the uterus is like the heart of a woman, because so many issues connected to our emotional hearts seem to revolve around the uterus—i.e., getting a period, not getting a period, being pregnant, not being pregnant, PMS, and menopause. It would follow that an affair of the heart might cause us to direct energies to the uterus, because it is sometimes difficult to talk about the pain, the sadness, the changes, or the loss. *Our body speaks to us when our minds can't.* (Many women with unusual bleeding are perimenopausal and so bleeding can be due to the lessening of hormones. However, relationship issues seem linked to bleeding, and often perimenopausal women are going through relationship changes—divorce, children growing up, second marriages, changing careers, or any lifestyle transition that involves changing roles.)

One patient of mine, for example, was in her 40s and thus perimenopausal when her husband abruptly left her. She stopped having periods. She did not feel that she was menopausal, even though she had no periods after the sudden end of her marriage. My feeling was that the shock to her system affected her hypothalamus functioning (the hypothalamus in the brain is involved in hormone production), and that is why she suddenly became menopausal.

In another instance, a patient's divorce seemed to stop her periods completely. She wanted to know if she was genuinely menopausal, or just overstressed. I drew her blood for a Follicle Stimulating Hormone (FSH) test, which tells us if a woman is menopausal. The result was above 35, which meant that she was menopausal. She chose to begin hormone replacement therapy. A year later she came back and said, "I really wonder if I'm menopausal. I may not be, and if I'm not, I could still get pregnant." We did another FSH, and this time it was under 35. She was now in a much better situation, she was calmer, and she had adjusted to the divorce and was feeling good about herself. A lot of her stress had been eliminated. She was apparently no longer menopausal, which meant that perhaps she never was truly in menopause to begin with. Her divorce confused her hormones so much that she tested menopausal. After one year on hormone replacement therapy, we switched her to birth control pills so she wouldn't get pregnant.

This patient had the intuition that she was not menopausal, and as we talked, I realized that she had some inner sense about it. We should not give short shrift to these inner messages, nor forget that the mind and the body are one.

As I mentioned at the beginning of this book, I had melanoma many years ago at the start of my career, so my recent experience with basal cell carcinoma was not the first time I have had to confront my own codependent leanings. When I developed the early melanoma (a skin cancer that can spread to vital organs), I was in what I feel was another codependent relationship. My thoughts were always centered on my husband and what he was doing, his career, and his needs. I was working full time, commuting long distances daily, managing two houses, and handling it "all." I began to realize how unhappy I was, and that I was depressed by it "all." It truly scared me to think I could die of this condition. I was forced, back against the wall, to look my own codependency in the eye. Ever since then, I have tried to be *honest* with myself about my feelings and relationships. I talk about my anger in twelve-step programs and therapy, so that it's not a secret or a surprise to me. I try to speak up about what I want and need. I learned to listen to my body. The melonoma told me everything I needed to know. Years later, the basal cell carcinoma told me again. (I needed a reminder.)

Codependency sometimes seems like a cancer of the mind and soul. As Steven Locke and Douglas Colligan explain in *The Healer Within*, doctors have studied behavior patterns of melanoma patients and found many of them to be excessively nice, extremely compliant, and often passive.[14] Psychologist Lydia Temoshok found these patients in general did not express anger, fear or sadness, and she called this a Type C personality. Her research suggested that the way these patients handled some of their feelings—not expressing them—could affect whether the disease spreads or abates. Many of the patients who suffered relapses exhibited this Type C personality. Borysenko's research has demonstrated how the stress of suppressing emotions can produce less interferon, an anti-cancer substance produced by the Killer T cells.[15] My own personal experience certainly supports these findings.

Although all illness is not related to codependency, I firmly believe that some illnesses are. We don't diagnose symptoms as "codependency-related illness" because it's not an area that has been studied or validated a great deal. I have seen people in twelve-step recovery programs with physical illness and as they start to talk about their addiction, then to address their problems, and to take responsibility instead of *blaming* others for everything, their physical symptoms disappear and they get better. This is a self-care plan, something not often addressed in a typical medical office visit. Indeed, the link between illness and codependency is rarely or never addressed in a typical office visit.

As women, we are fortunate that we're nurturing, and that we have estrogen and progesterone to give us our feminine ways. But I believe we also need to focus on ourselves and what our needs are and what our bodies are trying to say to us. We deceive ourselves when we believe that the inner voice and intuition are unimportant. So many women invalidate their own experience, intuition, and feelings *as if they don't exist.* When I ask patients, "What do you think is going on? What is your body telling you?" they always know, and they are always surprised that they know. It's as if they know the answers, but they need permission to say it out loud. The answers are not outside ourselves. When we stop our codependent thinking, we recover that inner voice and listen to our bodies.

Shhhh . . . listen to yourself.

—5—

Illnesses of the Breast

Rita came to my office with a breast lump that had been there for over a year. I suggested she have it examined by a surgeon, but she didn't want to. It was quite round and symmetrical, but did not show up on a mammogram. One year later, she came back, and by this time the lump was irregular. I knew it was malignant. She was not concerned about it, but her husband had insisted that she see me. She kept telling me there was "nothing wrong." She finally agreed to a mammogram, but she still would not see a surgeon. This time, the mammogram showed an irregular mass that was most likely malignant. I finally persuaded her to see a surgeon, and he removed the malignant lump the next day.

Was Rita not listening to her intuition when she told me "nothing is wrong," or was she in what could have been called "fatal denial"?

Emotions Run High: Attitudes and Fears

No woman wants to hear there is "something wrong" with her breasts, and this has been true even when the woman died as a result. Cultural burdens about breasts (and the possibility of losing them) taint our thinking. Historically, large breasts predominate primitive images of fertility. This has not changed in the last ten thousand years, only now it's called "sexy" instead of "fertility." In ancient times, breasts symbolized nature's abundance and nurturing qualities, but in our culture the nurturing metaphor has become confused. Women are now supposed to care without cease, giving and

caretaking, endlessly and selflessly. Women have also traditionally engaged in low-paying professions and volunteer work,
where they are pervasively devalued relative to men, and of
course, there's no pay for motherhood.

Breast cancer can strike many kinds of women. However,
gynecologist Christiane Northrup, in her book *Women's Bodies, Women's Wisdom,* posits again that women's repressed
anger about life issues can lead to breast disease.[1] Northrup has
observed that many women with breast cancer are self-
sacrificing, inhibited sexually, and unable to accept help. They
hide their anger and hostility behind a pleasant veneer that
masquerades the truth. Some studies have also suggested that
certain cancer patients are Type C personalities, for whom
everything is "okay," even when it's not.[2] In effect, their cells
get programmed to let trouble in the door and passively try to
smooth it over. They dare not rock the boat, they don't express
their anger, and the pressure of containment actually causes
the cell wall to weaken. Northrup argues that people must look
deep inside themselves to see what needs to heal, be expressed,
or changed, in order to achieve good health. We need to listen
to those inner messages.

Northrup has seen many women patients who are afraid to
touch or value their breasts. She encourages women to respect
their breasts and treat them as if they are special. Culturally,
breast type is another factor here. Women have been taught
that if they don't have a certain type of breast—big and firm—
they are not feminine or attractive, and that there is something
wrong. Most women do not have perfectly shaped, equal, up-
lifted breasts. Nonetheless, images implanted by the media
make perfect breasts tantamount to sexuality and romance. We

need to learn to love and accept our bodies for what they are, despite our "perfect breast" oriented society.

Author Louise Hay believes that breasts represent mothering and nurturing, and that physical problems, such as cysts, lumps, and soreness can result from over-mothering, over-protecting, overbearing attitudes.[3] She sees a need for balance in women's lives, so that both they and those they nurture can be free to live their own lives (unhampered by aging umbilical cords). An excellent work on the topic, *Dr. Susan Love's Breast Book*, recounts how breasts have traditionally been associated with nurturance and survival.[4] Nurturing, giving, love, and mothering are all intertwined with a woman's self-image, feelings about her femininity, motherhood issues, feeling misjudged, misunderstood, or not respected. If a woman can only give but not receive, there may be an imbalance leading to depletion of self; breasts are indicators of imbalance in our relationships.

Now when I talk about Hay's, Northrup's, and Love's theories, my physician friends especially always ask me, "Where's the scientific proof?"

I respond by relating the many conversations I have had with patients over the last 13 years. Often women who come in with symptoms (nipple discharge, a mass, or pain) are also feeling relationship stress. Their stories seem to validate the theories of Hay or Love: they feel pressured to take care of the whole world, or their mother has come to live with them, or they are ending a long-term relationship. Can it be coincidence that these events and breast symptoms occur simultaneously? If we are all connected by the same energy field (as the research of Dr. Larry Dossey and Dr. Deepak Chopra suggests), then I find it difficult to deny the connection between the relationships we are involved in, and the symbolism of the breasts.[5]

Women often feel relieved and validated when I explain there might be such a connection. They tell me it helps them to explain and understand what is happening. Recently a patient called because she had felt a lump in her breast, and she and I both felt instinctively it was malignant. Subsequent mammogram results suggested the lump was a nonmalignant cyst, but I did not believe it was a cyst, so I arranged for her to see a surgeon for a biopsy the next day. The biopsy proved the lump was indeed malignant, and when I talked to her, I explained some of the theories about possible connections between breast masses and relationships. She said she was not surprised, given what she had experienced in recent years— no love relationship, job demotion, and a bout with Lyme's Disease—an infectious condition she got from the bite of a deer tick. She definitely felt that there was a mind-body connection at work.

In the early 1970s, when I was working with tumor specialist Dr. Irving Ariel, a surgeon/oncologist at the Pack Medical Foundation in New York, I saw a great many breast cancer patients who were diagnosed late. By the time they came to us, they needed radical treatment. I began to look at cancer differently—I no longer wanted to be just putting out fires. I began to wonder a lot about the *beginning* of the disease, not just the *end.* I wondered why some people get sick and other people don't. Why did some women develop breast cancer at certain points in their lives? I read books on nutrition, psychology, and the mind/body connection, and talked to patients over and over. I began to view the role of holistic health as paramount to physical health. The mind and the body cannot be separated, and where breasts are concerned, fear rules the day.

My experience has taught me that women don't examine their breasts because they are afraid of what they might find, or they think they don't know what they're doing, or that they don't know exactly what they are supposed to be looking for. In my office, I have a silicone model of a breast with masses in it, and I have women examine it so they can know what a mass feels like. They are surprised to discover what they feel in their own breasts is normal tissue, because the model masses feel so distinctly different; they have circumference and borders (regular or irregular) that make them palpable.

I also believe most women are more familiar with their own breasts than we practitioners are—a personal observation that *is* supported by research. At a breast cancer conference I attended, I learned about a University of North Carolina study of breast masses where only 40% of doctors involved were able to locate breast masses, and gynecologists as a group found even fewer masses.[6] Breast illness is not what some gynecology specialists keep current and knowledgeable about, because our focus is generally on the uterus, ovaries, and vagina. In my experience, among practitioners, surgeons are the most successful at locating breast masses. However, those best equipped to find breast masses are women themselves, because they become so familiar with their own bodies that they "just know" when something is not right. The researchers of that same study just mentioned found that 85% of women who developed breast cancer knew it before they were diagnosed, and in some cases knew it and couldn't convince the medical establishment.

During my tenure with Dr. Ariel, he conducted a 20-year follow-up study of women who had radical mastectomies. At the time, mastectomies were the only type of surgery being performed. His observations suggested that cure rates over 20 years were linked to early detection, *not* with type of treatment. Clearly, although women might be afraid to find "something wrong" during self-examination, it saves lives.[7]

Most of the work I do is getting people to trust their own knowledge of themselves. Some studies of mammogram use indicate that women either find their own breast masses, or just suspect that something is wrong, more often than mammograms do. One theory holds that it takes six years to actually palpate a mass, but a mammogram can detect it earlier.[8] Some findings are showing about 15% to 20% of mammograms are inaccurate, or that they miss breast masses in women under age 50, due to the density of younger women's tissue.[9] Although mammograms have gotten mixed reviews, they have great value insofar as they can detect a mass years earlier than an exam, and have thus saved women's lives. We just need to understand they are not 100% accurate. Women frequently locate their own masses, and can be cured if they avail themselves of early treatment.

During mammography, a woman is exposed to radiation equivalent to 5 "rads," which is 13 fewer rads than we are exposed to when flying in airplanes. New methods of locating breast lumps have been introduced, and now some X-rays are done from the back, which involves considerably fewer rads than a mammogram. Mammograms do not cause cancer (through their radiation), and if they detect a microscopic mass, it can generally be cured directly as a result of such early detection. I see many women whose cancer was cured because their lump was detected, by mammogram, so early that it was a microcalcification, a speck of calcium that looks like a tiny piece of dust on the mammogram. Microcalcifications are sometimes but not usually an indication of cancer. However, when they appear in a cluster together, then your surgeon will do a biopsy to determine whether they are benign or cancerous. Microcalcifications cannot be felt or seen except on a mammogram.[10]

Feelings about self-examination and getting a mammogram vary widely from individual to individual, and there are numerous ways to approach these issues.[11] The facts are these: *self-examination on a regular basis is an important tool to detect breast cancer early, but mammography is the most important tool because it gives us the greatest chance for a cure.*

The Straight Facts

I find that women are very aware of their own bodies, and even if they are not examining their own breasts, they know intuitively when something is wrong. They tell me, "I think something is there," or, "I had a dream and something is going on in my breast." Getting the facts always allays fear. I have one patient whose mother died of breast cancer, and every time she felt something she would become hysterically fearful. She would call me on the phone and could not stop crying. She needed to get all the facts before she could calm down. I sent her to a surgeon, and after a careful exam and mammogram, he reassured her that she was not dying or even sick. I gave her literature on "markers" for women with a family history of breast cancer, so she could decide whether she wanted to have that type of evaluation done. Studies now show that these "markers" in the breasts yield information about the probability of malignancy. These are valuable tests for women whose mothers or aunts had breast cancer.[12]

Breasts are composed of fat, breast tissue, arteries, veins, nerves, ducts, lobules (a type of lobe), connective tissue, glands, and muscle. When a breast has multiple cysts occurring throughout the muscles and tissue, it is called a "fibrocystic" breast. These cysts are tiny, numerous, and densely distributed. Some practitioners tell women, "Oh, you have cystic breasts." This is not cause for alarm (although it might mean the practitioner should brush up on bedside manner). Chances are, a great many of us do have cystic breasts, although women who have completely normal tissue are sometimes told they have cystic breasts. Often women are told they have lumpy breasts, and this frightens them. However, this "lumpiness" which they feel can, in fact, be normal breast tissue composed of all the above-listed parts.[13] It's important that women know this so they are not walking around thinking there is something "wrong" with their breasts. I am continuously told by patients that they were afraid they had breast disease, and felt relieved to hear that normal breast tissue sometimes feels "lumpy."

Breast illness and functions are affected by estrogen production, which is linked to the menstrual cycle. Many women develop fibrocystic deposits just prior to their menstrual periods, but they disappear as the period begins. When you examine your breasts, be aware of where you are in your menstrual cycle, if you still get periods. If you find masses (lumps) before your period, then examine them again after your period. My feeling is that women still produce estrogen even when they are menopausal. They may produce varying amounts, contingent upon how the adrenals are functioning, but you're always going to have some hormonal production. How much depends on how fit your adrenal glands are, what type of foods you are eating, how you're thinking about life, and handling stress. You could still have fibrocystic breast masses depending on hormonal production, even if you are menopausal.

Another type of breast mass is the fibroadenoma, a nonmalignant, benign mass. They are usually symmetrical, round, and firm, and they do not adhere or stick to the breast wall. You can move them around. However, because they are round and hard, it's difficult to tell whether they are malignant. Sometimes a mammogram will indicate some earmarks of malignancy, but we cannot always be sure. Most surgeons would recommend a biopsy. In all cases, we have to look at the combination of holistic and traditional approaches. You have to gather much information and make your own choices based on your own intuitive process, your inner wisdom. That's what we women need to learn to do.

Another type of breast mass is ductal ecstasia, which is a pre-cancerous condition. It usually occurs near the nipple and should be surgically removed so it doesn't become malignant. Many breast masses occur under the nipple, and most women don't examine under the nipple. The other place they are found in is the area which goes from the breast tissue up into the axilla (underarm). You need to examine under your arm, as well as the breast and the nipple.

Nipple inversion is often a symptom of cancer (assuming the woman is not one of a minority born with inverted nipples).

A nipple that has never been inverted can become so if an underlying breast mass pulls it in.

Inflammation is often symptomatic of abscesses of the breasts. In these cases, the nipple or some other area turns very red. Redness can also come about during pregnancy or breast feeding. There may be discharge from the nipple or from the inflamed area. Redness can also accompany cancer, so differential diagnosis is important. There are many different types of cancer, but most all of them are preceded by a mass that doesn't move, is irregular, or is not tender. Usually a malignant mass is not tender, except in the case of inflammatory breast cancer in its later stages. A slide (sample) of any discharge can be made to help in a diagnosis.

For instance, you might find enlarged lymph nodes under the armpit. There are lymph nodes that follow the internal mammary glands, which are in between the two breasts and also in the neck, and they can become enlarged. Lymph nodes are filtering systems whose role is to drive impurities out. This does not mean, if you have lymph nodes in your neck or armpit, that you have breast cancer. Each case is different and requires a review of all the facts. A professional examination should be done whenever there is doubt.

Over the past twenty years, practitioners have realized that lumpectomies are just as valid as mastectomies depending on the type size, and location of the tumor. Studies reveal that early detection and adequate removal (lumpectomy) of the cancer, coupled with changing diet and lifestyle, are very successful.[14] If you notice a breast mass, then consult a surgeon with whom you feel comfortable and who will listen to what you have to say. We need to advocate for ourselves in the matter of lumpectomy versus mastectomy. A patient–doctor relationship should be like a good marriage. If it's not, I always encourage women to find another practitioner with whom they can work. You may have to get many opinions before you get to the truth, *your truth.*

Holistic Approaches

The last twenty years of research on holistic health is quite definitive: you *can* change your life. There is a great deal to be said for the work we do on ourselves, and this is particularly true for bodily parts as fraught with emotions as breasts.

Do we inherit disease genetically, or do we inherit the *patterns* of our relatives? If we can shepherd even a fragment of change into those patterns—thinking patterns, eating patterns, lifestyle patterns—we will be able to change the outcome of disease through prevention. Ancient Chinese medical tenets hold that we exhibit certain energy patterns before we are born.[15] We start imitating our relatives' habits and diet in the womb because we have no choice—we have to eat what our mother eats. People who break the concrete wall of habit start by examining inherited behavior. Then they decide how they choose to live and eat and care for themselves, rather than blindly adopting the routine of their forebears. You can wedge novelty into the fortress of custom, but it takes conscious effort (particularly when Aunt Esther accosts you at a family reunion, crying, "You're not eating any of my fudge? I made it just for you!"). My experience has been that food is often not used for nourishment, but rather to suppress feelings, something many of us learned in our family of origin. A healthier response might be to talk about what you're feeling, rather than putting something into your mouth in order to suppress it. Let's consider, for example, the change in lifestyle that can be brought about by being honest with ourselves.

Psychoneuroimmunology suggests that people who feel their feelings, instead of suppressing them, may have an elevated immune response. If you claim to feel "fine" but are really ready to scream, you send your cells mixed messages. As a result, *something is going to go wrong somewhere between the mind and the cells.* In every cell is a receptor that conveys information about both the emotions you are experiencing but not expressing as well as the emotions you are experiencing and expressing openly.

Again according to Chinese medicine, cancer is thought to stem from unresolved issues, whether they be physically or emotionally painful to bear.[16] Imbalance between giving and receiving can lead to physical manifestations such as breast cysts and breast masses. We cannot just give to others, or just take from others—a balance must be struck between the two.[17] My belief is that the body is a balanced scale and if you have a symptom, that means something is out of balance in your life or in your environment. What that something is, is up to you to figure out.

Our bodies talk to us about lack of balance. When we feel anger, for example, we need to talk about it and to express it in a way that is appropriate. This does not mean kicking the cat or attacking the husband. Harriet Goldhor Lerner, author of *Dance of Anger,* describes how underneath anger is fear, sadness, or other issues.[18] We need to unearth what our anger is about. When it comes to breast cancer, there are clearly some things we can control and some things we can't. People seek out august medical authorities expecting answers, but it's not that simple. There are some things practitioners cannot figure out for us, and that we have to figure out for ourselves.

Prevention

Cultural dictates gear women to look for disease. The push for mammography is based upon the desire to *find* disease, not to protect against it. Few medical practitioners talk about diet, caring for your breasts, or loving your breasts. We repeatedly focus on getting sick and finding illness, instead of how we can prevent ourselves from getting sick.

When we don't take responsibility for our health, we presume we are victims of our ill health. If it's cancer, there's nothing we can do about it, except maybe catch it early. That's wrong. There is much that you can do. Cancer prevention is a daily affair. It's a matter of how you live your life.

Some studies now suggest that dietary fat may contribute to, but does not necessarily cause, breast cancer, while other studies still suggest that 27% of breast cancers are attributable to dietary fat.[19] Many theories hold that women who eat more fat produce more estrogen, and normal breast functions are adversely affected by the presence of too much estrogen. In addition, we may be ingesting high levels of estrogen because some of the meat, cheese, and milk in our diets comes from animals that have been fed hormones. Not eating sufficient fiber can cause us to retain these hormones as well as other toxins, which build up in the bowel and then lower the immune response. Radiation has also been linked to breast cancer and studies are indicating that women who live close to radioactive fallout sites have a peculiarly high incidence of breast cancer.[20]

What are we to do? We can minimize our risks of breast cancer by lowering our fat intake, eating more fiber in order to eliminate toxins, and becoming proactive about radioactive dumping. There is no one, sure, rubber-stamp method of preventing breast cancer, but I believe the more active we become in wellness, the more we may reduce our risks.

Diet, lifestyle, stress, trauma—all these things are on the list of predisposing factors. Alcohol is a predisposing factor linked with breast cancer.[21] Alcohol suppresses the immune response and also the emotions, so drinking women won't express what they honestly feel. Alcohol makes us express all sorts of things, but are they appropriate and are they real? If the cells are awash in alcohol and numb because of it, they cannot see invaders, and the immune system becomes suppressed. Cigarettes also suppress the immune response.[22] Nicotine is a major addiction, and it's even often compared to heroin. Avoiding alcohol and nicotine is one way to decrease the risk of breast cancer.

Sugar can also depress the immune system, and this makes the body more susceptible to all disease, including breast cancer.[23] There are steps we can take to help reduce our craving for, and to stop eating, sugar. Herbalists can suggest many herbs that reduce sugar craving and balance the blood sugar. Chromium, available in capsule form, homeopathic sugars, and

B vitamins are often recommended for sugar withdrawal.[24] The more complex carbohydrates you eat, the more your craving for sugar goes down. *Craving for sugar indicates a lack of balance in nutrition.*

Bioflavonoids, found in green and orange vegetables, as well as in beans, can increase the production of protective enzymes in the tissues and also reduce excessive activity of estrogen.[25]

Bioflavonoids are found in citrus fruits, grapes, plums, black currants, apricots, buckwheat, cherries, and blackberries.[26] Carotenes and bioflavinoids are related to each other. Vegetables are the primary source of good things in the diet. The cruciferous vegetables—fibrous ones like cabbage, broccoli, kale, or anything in the cabbage family—change the way estrogen is synthesized. They also act as fiber, so again they are eliminating unhealthy elements from the bowel. Selenium, also found in vegetables, is an anti-oxidant which destroys unwanted toxins. Antioxidants are vital to our immune systems. Foods high in phyto-estrogens, for example, foods made from soybeans (tofu, miso, tempeh) also may help prevent breast cancer.[27] This may be one of the reasons Japanese women have such a low incidence of breast cancer, since they eat minimal animal fats and many soy products.[28] Linoleic acid oils (primrose, borage, or black currant) may reduce the incidence of breast masses and possibly even breast cancer.[29]

Waiting until you get a diagnosis of breast illness is not the time to decide what you want to do. When your back is against the wall, in this culture, it takes a special and unusual kind of person to be able to embrace holistic medicine. It also takes health care providers who are willing to give you support. So I tell my patients to start eliminating toxins, and using herbs, good nutrition, vitamins, and stress reduction *now,* not later.

Currently, one out of every ten women develops breast cancer.[30] That is a staggeringly high percentage, but it can be lowered and prevented if we maintain optimal wellness, be true to ourselves, and listen to our bodies.

—6—

Sexuality and Sexually Transmitted Diseases

Sarah was in her seventies and suffering greatly from heart ailments. Her daughter, Josie, trucked her to a variety of heart specialists, at prodigious expense to both their bank accounts, but Sarah continued to deteriorate. One day, while struggling gamely to eat lunch despite her disabilities, Sarah met Joseph at the nursing home where she lived. Neither Sarah nor Joseph had model figures, silky complexions, or what you might call sex appeal. But they did have camaraderie, and eventually quite a yen for each other. They started having sex and Sarah's heart symptoms disappeared. Indeed, she enjoyed better health than she had for fifteen years.

Despite the fact that Sarah's heart improved and symptoms began to disappear, Josie thought she would die of embarrassment when discreetly informed of the situation. She was disgusted and ashamed of her mother, even though it was obvious that sex had helped to save her mother's life.

The Taboo of Talking about It

Like Josie, most of us don't accept that our parents have or had sex, even though we clearly wouldn't exist if they hadn't. *Sex* is something we hear a great deal about, joke endlessly about, and assume that we're sophisticated about—something marketing firms all use to their advantage. But when it comes to the bottom line, very few talk honestly about sex. How does this implicitly agreed-upon societal pact affect our health? We know that keeping secrets hurts our spiritual health, and sooner or later that will affect our physical health. Unfortunately, medical professionals (other than psychologists) usually don't query patients about sex and rarely consider it a part of wellness. How many practitioners ever asked you about your sex life? Would you have been embarrassed if they did? Would your practitioners likely have been embarrassed, too? Patients rarely ever get to talk about the effect of sex on health. It's as if we try to pretend we are not sexual beings, or it's just too uncomfortable to discuss. Sexuality, however, is related to health in countless ways.

When we do sexuality counseling, *we give people permission,* we give them learning, we give them information, and we provide them with a safe, non-threatening place to talk. What most people need is permission to discuss taboo subjects. Once they have information, they can address many situations themselves. Half the problem is lack of sound information. I give my patients books to read, and then we talk about what is happening in their lives. They need to be validated, and to know their experience is not a product of their imaginations. I try to provide a safe place for women to ask any questions they want, and to not feel embarrassed or censored. What better place for this to occur than a women's health care office?

For example, many women are anorgasmic (they don't have orgasms) and have been either too embarrassed to mention it or they feel abnormal. They seem to feel safe in my office since I try to be non-judgmental, real, accepting, and an equal of theirs. They feel *validated* when they find out there are many other women with similar concerns, and that this is not unusual or abnormal and can be handled rather easily with proper information and techniques.

How do we learn about sexuality?—down behind the barn, in some traditions. We learn from friends, older siblings, relatives, magazines, or movies. We learn subliminally from our parents, because if you witnessed your parents touching, hugging, kissing, and communicating as a result, you might on some level have perceived that being sexual is a part of living. One of the most effective ways of communicating is sexually, if it's an appropriate communication. Couples who do not communicate sexually are not communicating on other levels either.[1] If you grow up watching parents abuse each other verbally or physically, or with few or no expressions of sexuality, unhealthy messages about sex may have been passed on to you.

Taboos concerning sex talk are intergenerational. Many women come to my office asking me to see their daughters, talk to them about sexuality, and tell them not to have sex. They hope that "someone else"—a practitioner, a teacher, a coach—will discuss what they perceive themselves as incapable of doing. Parents are woefully faint-hearted about their adult responsibilities, about children losing innocence, and about the use of protection. Often the young daughters are comfortable with their own sexuality, but the parents think they need education or a physical exam. Some parents want their daughters to have information and to protect themselves, and are sensitive to the fact that young people might be more comfortable talking to a professional rather than to a parent. If a girl has made the choice to be sexually active, she needs protection such as birth control pills, a diaphragm, a cervical cap, condoms, or other barrier methods. Contrary to some public opinions, we do not make our children sexually active by keeping them informed and protected. The more information they receive, the more appropriate are their choices. Although they may be uncomfortable verbalizing it, parents know that adolescents who have much information do make good choices for themselves. It is indeed the adolescents without information who encounter trouble. Children who are sexually active and promiscuous at a young age are often looking for love, or perhaps capitulating to peer pressure—two topics parents are reluctant to admit and discuss.

Often, both the parent and the child want to talk about sexuality, but don't know how or when to start the dialogue. In adolescence, too, sudden, disruptive change is commonplace: one minute teens are adults, and the next they are little children. It can unravel the best-adjusted parent. Teens can be adult about sexuality or they can behave like children. Adolescent thinking also tends toward denial, as in "nothing will ever happen to me." Another reason parents have trouble talking to children is that at the time adolescents are dealing with sexual identity and awakenings they are thirteen, fourteen, or fifteen. This puts parents in their late thirties or forties. Parents may be having their own mid-life crises which can involve their own sexual questions (who am I, what do I want, and where have I been?). If parents have not dealt with their own sexuality, they will predictably clam up when confronted with a "budding" teenager. Thus an unwillingness to discuss sexuality is passed from generation to generation, which is unfortunate because sexual honesty is critical to healing sexual disease, right from the beginning. This legacy has led to a situation where, although people are now more open about sexuality than they used to be, clouds of shyness still swirl about. Talking propels our (and our parents') uneasiness into a spotlight. Our early memories and impressions of sex imprint our present behavior. People who have been sexually abused often have problems in relationships, and these women can have great difficulties with gynecological exams. Some women die of uterine or breast cancer, because they would rather die than have a doctor touch them. Why are we embarrassed to death about sex and health?

Sex and Health

Sexual activity can stimulate hormone production, the adrenal glands, and the heart rate, which lowers the stress response.[2] A lowered stress response improves immune response. Studies have shown that people who are sexually active have low levels of pain in illness and a general feeling of well being because of the hormone stimulation.[3]

Sexuality has been shown to be a valuable treatment for psychological problems, as long as it's appropriate sexuality.[4] We are not talking here about having ten partners at once or forcing others to have sex. Appropriate sex pumps up the entire endocrine system so that it works better, and a smoothly flowing endocrine system enhances the immune system. Cardiovascular health is improved by sex.[5] Some research has linked healthy sex with smoother skin, preventing depression, and slowing certain aging processes.[6] Sexually active women produce more estrogen, so their menstrual cycles are more regular.[7] Orgasm activates endorphins, sometimes resulting in less severe PMS, and it can also relieve insomnia and promote general relaxation.[8] In this respect, sexuality can be healing to the immune system.

This could explain why so many more sonnets, odes, symphonies, and songs are written about love and its effects than, say, doing taxes or folding the wash.

In his "Needs Hierarchy," psychologist Abraham Maslow reasoned that we have to satisfy certain basic needs to live.[9] The first need is for air to breathe, and the second need is for food to eat. The third need is for shelter from the elements, and the fourth need is sexuality. We must satisfy the first three needs before attending to the fourth. Maslow postulates that if you satisfy these basic needs, you can then go to the next level of hierarchy, which is self-actualization. Self-actualization is the highest level of meeting needs. Self-actualization means doing what really makes you happy, evolving to the highest place you can be in life and the world. Those who make a commitment to something bigger than themselves are often the most self-actualized.

My work with menopausal women demonstrates Maslow's theory. For those women who have a commitment to goals, and who have activities in their lives that they feel are important contributions, transit through menopause is much less painful. Adolescents with goals also see fewer struggles in terms of teenage pregnancies, sexuality, and sexually transmitted diseases.

Michael Carrera, a sexuality educator, theorizes that if teenagers have goals they are less likely to get pregnant or to contract sexually transmitted diseases.[10] His work is timely, considering the high rate of AIDS among teenagers. Carrera works with inner city families to help parents create goals for themselves and their children. He has been instrumental in obtaining college scholarships, grants, and jobs for at-risk teens and their parents as well. Carrera's work reveals that when children see their parents having goals, getting back into school or working at a career they enjoy, then the teenagers have hope. They see there is something they can do with life, and this also decelerates the rate of teenage suicide. When their parents have goals, teens have higher aspirations themselves, and better feelings about what their future might be. Goals motivate them to take better care of themselves sexually. They use protection to avoid disease and pregnancy, because they have a reason to live. If you want to live, you are less likely to be having sex with many partners, drinking, or drugging. Holistically speaking, if you heal whatever is underneath that creates sadness, depression, or need, then you do not engage in behavior that lowers the immune response.

How we perceive sexual health can affect what transpires inside the body. Sensations permeate sexuality and we need to be aware of them. Anxiety can wrap around our every cell when it comes to sex. Was my first message about sex a good message or a bad message? Do I want to change the message? Do I want to change it for my children, or the people in my life? Childhood conditioning remains in force unless or until we peel it off. Do we see ourselves as sexual beings, as healthy sexual beings, or as bundles of shame? Current problems with sexuality in a relationship may be based on deep-seated memories. Joan Borynsenko, author of *Guilt Is the Teacher, Love Is the Lesson,* is a psychoneuroimmunologist who guides people to heal their original pain by talking about it, revealing it, not hushing it up.[11] People who hold on to bad memories or childhood traumas may also have fewer Killer T cells, whereas people who let go of pain may see their Killer T cell level rise.

Perhaps this explains why practitioners see so many sexually abused individuals develop illnesses.

Aging and Sex

Let's debunk a useless old myth, the one that says it is not okay to be sexual as we age. There's an unspoken adage that as we age we are not sexual beings, or we shouldn't be, or we shouldn't talk about it if we are. Older people often have the need or desire, but are too embarrassed to say so because they have bought into the myth. Why are aging couples, people who have lived together all their lives, put into separate rooms in nursing homes? Their sexuality may be confined to touching and being close, yet they are denied even that. What does this do to their minds and their health, once they are deprived of a connection that is important to them? I believe it could hasten their demise, or at least cause them to shut down emotionally.

In terms of health, we should never forget that sexuality is part of our being. It also seems quite unfair for others to arbitrarily decide that the elderly, for instance, are no longer sexual beings. Sexual and orgasmic response are slower with age, but not absent altogether. If partners can be patient, and if they receive accurate information about pace from their health care practitioners, then they themselves can choose whether or not they are sexual beings. What happens so often in the case of elderly patients is that they stop talking about or even having sex because they are embarrassed or uncomfortable, or they think they shouldn't, or couldn't, but in most cases they can, and if they want to, then they should. As healers, we practitioners need to maintain an open mind on the subject by dealing with our own feelings about sexuality, so that people are not embarrassed to come to us. Sexuality is important to health and healing. "Sexuality" does not mean only vigorous intercourse, although it is entirely possible to have sexual relations late in life. Sexuality means how people perceive themselves, how they walk and talk, how they interact with others. Sexuality can mean holding hands in the case of elderly persons too physically infirm to engage in intercourse.

Sexually Transmitted Diseases

Avoiding Sexually Transmitted Disease (STD) underlies and supports a healthy sex life, which means taking responsibility for loving ourselves and caring for ourselves. It means being reasonable and adult in our thinking and approach to sex. It means respecting ourselves enough to want to avoid STD or venereal disease. "Venereal" means transmitted by sexual intercourse, and reasonableness means using protection, which is usually a condom. This applies unless we are in a long-term monogamous relationship, where both partners have tested negative for STDs. Monogamous means neither we nor our partners are having sex with anyone else, and that means *absolutely*. We need to ensure that we can trust our partners, and that our wildly throbbing hearts are not shutting our love-blinded eyes to the truth about whether our partners are monogamous or not. In this age of AIDS, to swallow a half-truth hook, line, and sinker can be fatal. The holistic approach means taking responsibility for our own life, sometimes despite the perfumed enchantment of candle-light and promises.

If we experience symptoms of STD, a prompt visit to a medical practitioner can be life-saving.

Chlamydia is now recognized as a leading STD, more common than gonorrhea. Chlamydia causes pain on urination, a yellow or sometimes greenish discharge, itching, pelvic pain, and/or pain during intercourse or during a pelvic exam. Often the infection is not painful despite minor inflammation of the pelvic organs. Men will often have symptoms before their female partners do, and women can feel well until the infection reaches the uterus. A large percentage of women may have asymptomatic and therefore undetected chlamydia. Although women may not be aware of its presence, men usually do have symptoms of discharge and burning on urination. Chlamydia infections can cause pelvic inflammatory disease or, if undetected for a long time, infertility or infection of a newborn's eyes during a vaginal birth.

If the partner is not treated, chlamydia can be passed back and forth without the (nonsymptomatic) woman partner realizing it. Open communication, truth, and honesty with a partner about possible symptoms is of paramount importance to the early detection of chlamydia. Prescription antibiotics are the usual treatment, with both partners being treated before resuming intercourse. Zithromax in one substantial dose, or Floxin or Doxycline twice a day for 7 days, are the usual recommendations.

Gonorrhea, another common STD, can infect the uterus, fallopian tubes, and ovaries. In its early stages, it can be unnoticeable. Some women will experience painful or frequent urination. Stomach pain and fever accompany the advance of gonorrhea. Conventional antibiotic treatment relieves symptoms and cures gonorrhea. However, if the infection has gone unchecked for a substantial time, infertility can result. Again, both partners must be treated. A simple test called the Gen-Probe, which is inserted into the cervix, can detect chlamydia and gonorrhea.

Trichomonas, a parasite, can be sexually transmitted. The symptoms resemble those of chlamydia and gonorrhea—pelvic pain, pain on urination or with intercourse, or a yellow frothy discharge with a fishy odor. Like some other STDs, it is entirely curable but can cause infertility if not diagnosed and treated. Professional examination is necessary to discern whether an infection is actually trichomonas, and not chlamydia or gonorrhea. Trichomonas can be detected in an office visit, using what is called a "wet mount" with a microscope, or by doing a Pap smear. A woman might have a malodorous discharge or pain during the exam, resulting from an inflamed cervix or uterine tenderness.

Trichomonas is treated with the prescription item Flagyl, which seems to work the best. I prescribe 2 grams of Flagyl (4 tablets) on a one-time basis *for both partners,* then check them both post-treatment. Sometimes one dose is curative, but not always. If *both* partners are not cured, I prescribe 250 mg. 3 times a day for a week.

There are two kinds of *Herpes:* Herpes Simplex and Herpes Zoster. Herpes Zoster is related to chicken pox and causes shingles. In my practice, I more commonly see Herpes Simplex. Herpes Simplex One occurs on the mouth, while Herpes Simplex Two occurs on the vulva, but they are both exactly the same virus. An open draining lesion (clear fluid) on the mouth or a painful draining lesion on a woman's vagina or cervix, or on the man's penis, is one sign of Herpes.

Fever blisters on the mouth are Herpes Simplex lesions. Practitioners label mouth lesions "Herpes One" and genitalia lesions "Herpes Two." If your immune system is in exuberant shape, you may not experience recurrences, but when stress or diet or other interferences deplete the immune system, blisters recur. If you had fever blisters as a child, the virus remains in your body. If you have oral sex and either partner has a fever blister on the mouth, then Herpes can be transmitted to the genitals. If you have Herpes on your genitals and somebody has oral sex with you, they can get it on their mouth.

The fluid from the genital lesions is clear and especially painful during urination. I advise people to try to pour water over their genitals during urination because if urine passes over the lesions it slows down healing, not to mention stinging beyond description. Sometimes enlarged lymph nodes in the groin area will also be a sign of Herpes.

People usually know if they have Herpes. I come out of my office to greet them in the waiting room, and they are standing because they cannot sit down. People are so often surprised by this disease, and they want to know where they got it. The reason Herpes can be sexually transmitted is that it is a virus, skin-to-skin contact occurs during sex (or kissing, in the case of a mouth lesion), and liquid virus draining from the lesion passes into the other person's pores.

Herpes is also communicable during what is called its "podromal" phase, which occurs just prior to an outbreak of lesions. Symptoms of this phase are tingling or burning in the genital area. Herpes is not communicable once the lesion has disappeared completely. People with Herpes need to talk it over with their partners and to practice safe sex by using condoms until the lesions have disappeared. I know people in long-term relationships where one person has Herpes and the other has never contracted it. There are two reasons this happens: first, they practice safe sex during outbreaks, and second, the non-infected partner could have such a competent immune system that he or she will never get the virus.

I receive many frantic telephone calls about Herpes. Women are in an outrage. How did they get this? They are sure they got it from their partners, who may not have been forth-right about symptoms. Men will tell me the woman gave it to them because they never had it before. Patients and their partners want to know where it came from; however, medicine does not have all the answers at this time. Many practitioners I speak to suspect that a large percentage of the population has latent Herpes, and we are not certain how it is contracted since it is not always sexually transmitted.[12] It is possible that any one of us can experience an outbreak at any point in our lives, and this is particularly true when we are under stress. I once heard a story about a doctor who had been married for twenty-five years, was monogamous, and never had Herpes. On the day of his wife's funeral, he had a terrible outbreak. He could not imagine how he had contracted Herpes. My suspicion is that it had been in his body for years, and the outbreak occurred because the grief of losing a beloved partner lowered his immune response. Although it can and does go into remission, Herpes is not curable. Whether or not you have an outbreak sometimes depends on how you take care of yourself.

The conventional treatment is to apply the prescription item Zovirax ointment to the lesions five times a day during the initial outbreak. If subsequent outbreaks occur, Zovirax capsules can be taken by mouth five times a day for five days, and from the moment you experience the first symptom, which can speed recovery. For patients who experience chronic outbreaks, I prescribe the capsules.

In holistic terms, Herpes can be treated by applying Listerine to the lesions. This is painful but they do dry right up. You also can apply Gentian Violet to lesions. This is an old, herbal remedy available at health food stores and pharmacies. Taking colossal amounts of acidophilus by mouth (five capsules every two hours) will speed up healing. Lots of Vitamin C, Vitamin B, and drinking water can hasten recovery. The goal is to flush the body of toxins and simultaneously elevate the immune system. Lysine, an amino acid available in capsule form, can be taken daily, in addition to acidophilus and vitamins, and this sometimes prevents or minimizes future attacks.[13] Again, decreasing alcohol, cigarettes, and stress may also prevent recurrence.[14]

Hepatitis B and *Hepatitis C* can be sexually transmitted as well. Fatigue is the primary symptom, with jaundice, brownish urine and yellow bowel movements. Hepatitis B and C are communicable through IV needles, as well as sexually, as is AIDS. Hepatitis B is now preventable with a vaccine. Vaccination is required for any hospital or health care facility employee, due to the high incidence of exposure, and is recommended for anyone in a relationship with someone with acute or chronic Hepatitis B. The vaccine is administered once a month for two months, and then once more six months later. Hepatitis B is not curable, but 90% of patients do see it depart into remission. The other 10% have chronically elevated liver enzymes, leaving them more prone to cirrhosis and liver cancer, because their liver is consistently inflammated.

The *Human Papilloma Virus* (HPV) is also called the *wart virus* or venereal wart, because it is a type of wart. It can be sexually transmitted, but not always. Scientists are not sure exactly how the wart virus is transmitted in all cases. It may originate in stress or some other psychoneuroimmunological factors, or it may result from environmental toxins. It is most commonly transmitted through sexual intercourse. Women who have warts on their vagina can be treated in the office with Podophyllin or Trichlorocetic Acid (TCA) applied directly to the lesions. After repeated applications at weekly intervals, the lesions are eliminated. Some women develop lesions on the cervix or in the endocervical canal. Such lesions are often only detected on a Pap smear but these are treated differently as we will discuss.

In a *small* percentage of women, certain types of HPV can predispose to cervical cancer—this is why yearly Pap smears with early detection are so important. I recommend a Pap every six months if a woman has had or been exposed to HPV. I have treated women with the wart virus, which untreated can lead to a pre-cancerous cervical lesion or even to cervical cancer. Women can be treated as outpatients with cryo-surgery (freezing off the cells that are not normal), a Loop Electrical Surgical Excision Procedure, known as LEEP (excision of the HPV cells from the endocervical canal, which means going into the cervical canal and scooping out any wart virus), or cone biopsy if detected early enough. They are not entirely cured in the typical sense of the word because the virus lives in the body forever in the immune system. The most we hope for is that it stays in remission. When women come to me with recurrent wart virus, I discuss immune system functioning with them. I ask them, "Are you smoking?" They are often smoking a pack of cigarettes a day. "Are you drinking?" Usually they are cocktail fans, and not just on weekends. Or, they are under stress they cannot cope with, and they are not doing anything about it. That is, they are not practicing stress reduction techniques. I encourage them to stop smoking and drinking, and to take lots of Vitamin C. Sometimes taking 400 mcg. of folic acid per day can deter recurrence of the wart virus. B vitamins and good food also lead to remission.

I often observe that in women burdened with stress the HPV makes an appearance. These women won't have had it for years, or they have never had it before, and when life railroads them they are in my office asking, "How did I get this?" When people do not understand causative factors here, a terrific strain is placed upon relationships. I have also seen couples break up over HPV occurrence, because they don't understand this virus can pop up at any point in their lives, as a direct function of how *well* they are—or are not. The wart virus may not have been transmitted by their present partner, and may not even be sexually transmitted. I recommend that all partners be checked for the wart virus since lesions can be unnoticeable to the naked eye; people can be HPV carriers without even knowing it. It would be senseless to treat a woman with HPV and not treat her partner who could be a potential source of transmission. Men can be checked by either a urologist or a dermatologist who is familiar with HPV detection. Treatment can be done on an outpatient basis, but, as with women, HPV will continue to live in a man's immune system even though it has been treated locally.

The presence of the Pap or wart virus in women is detected by the Pap test, or Pap smear. When a Pap smear comes back from lab analysis labeled positive, showing dysplasia or CIN (cervical intraepithelial neoplasia—a pre-cancerous lesion) the woman needs a colposcopy. This procedure magnifies our view of the cervix thirty times. The practitioner puts iodine on the cervix, and this causes anything suggestive of the virus, or an abnormality, to show up. A biopsy is done next. The biopsy takes about ten days to analyze. If it is positive for dysplasia or CIN, the woman is advised to have laser surgery, cryo-surgery, or a LEEP procedure. If the virus has travelled up into the cervix or uterus, a surgical cone biopsy is performed: a cone-shaped portion of the cervix being removed (conization). If not treated with either conization, LEEP, or cryo-surgery, the viral infection can progress to cancer of the uterus. In that case, hysterectomy (removal of the uterus) is recommended.

I have seen cervical cancer spread to the uterus only twice in the eleven years of my practice. Both women had similar situations. One woman had not had a Pap smear for three years. She had a great deal of bleeding but still had to be persuaded to come in for an exam. By the time I saw her she had a mass protruding from her cervix. She had radical surgery, but eventually she died. If she had had regular, yearly Pap smears, we could have cured her cancer with minor procedures. Cervical cancer is curable if detected early, and if it has not spread into vital organs.

The other woman had not had a Pap smear for fourteen years. She claimed to be practicing holistic medicine and to be concerned about wellness, but she was kidding herself in that department. Holistic health care in no way negates regular exams and testing—in fact, regular check-ups are critical to holistic medicine. She went to a practitioner in a great deal of pelvic pain and a CAT scan revealed a malignancy in her pelvis. During surgery, it was apparent the cancer had also spread to her bladder. Her ovaries, uterus, fallopian tubes and part of her bladder were removed, and she lived. This radical surgery might have been avoided if she had had routine yearly Pap smears. I cannot stress enough the importance of annual Pap smears. It is part of maintaining sexual health.

Sexually active women can have less PMS, fewer migraine headaches, elevated endorphin levels, and elevated hormone levels.[15] Does this occur for purely technical reasons, or does it evoke the power of the human connection? We are not quite sure how it all works, but sexuality is a robust force within the human body. Again, it's always important to be aware of what you're eating, how you're exercising, and what dynamic is at work in your relationships, but it is imperative to talk about what is happening to you sexually. We need to ask the pointed questions, and to seek out the healthy answers. Our lives depend on it.

—7—

Pre-Menstrual
Syndrome (PMS)

Pre-menstrual Syndrome, commonly known as PMS, affects a woman's life in myriad ways. There is more misinformation than information floating around about why and how this is so. Many women experiencing PMS are lead to believe it is "all in their heads." I believe PMS occurs due to hormone imbalances, which cause measurable, biochemical shifts in the bloodstream. It's not all in a woman's head.

Throughout a typical healthy menstrual cycle, estrogen and progesterone are produced in fluctuating levels, and are lower than average just prior to a period, causing pre-menstrual syndrome. After the period, these hormones start to build up, and at about mid-cycle they peak, causing ovulation. After ovulation, from mid-cycle on, both the estrogen and progesterone hormones start to drop again, which seems to be the time when women begin experiencing symptoms. The best way to know when PMS is beginning is to chart the symptoms as they surface. The biological effects of hormonal fluctuation are manifested as physical symptoms, exactly the same as any other biological fluctuation will be manifested as physical symptoms.

PMS symptoms can include nervousness, irritability, fatigue, breast tenderness, emotionalism, bloating, and general mood swings. Many women tell me they just feel "off the wall" and unusually intolerant. At another time of the month, something could happen and it wouldn't bother them at all, and then before their period some complain that they get irrational and it scares them. Women have also told me that their experiences with the traditional medical establishment have not been as they would wish in regard to PMS. Support and understanding, not superciliousness or disinterest, are vital here. It's also not unusual for physical difficulty to accompany hormonal imbalances. If a patient suffers an imbalance of hormones affecting the thyroid, we give them medication to correct the imbalance and relieve the symptoms. We don't tell them it's all in their heads. In the 1950s, Dr. Katarina Dalton, a British physician, became one of the first and few to scrutinize biochemical changes that occur during pre-menses, but since then little additional research has focused on PMS.[1]

Stress reduction plays a part here as well. At the Institute of HeartMath in Boulder Creek, California, researcher Rollin McCraty tracked 50 subjects for three months to determine the effects of stress reduction techniques on hormonal and immune systems.[2] Subjects' emotional states were measured daily, and blood was drawn to correlate emotional states with hormone levels. Subjects were also trained in stress reduction techniques designed to combat anger with more peaceful reactions to daily stress. People who were angry found that they could reduce their feelings of anger by use of various relaxation techniques. After two months, McCraty found that when his subjects were able to derail their anger somewhat and reported feeling less anxious, their blood hormone levels shifted. The presence of the stress hormone cortisol was reduced substantially. All subjects reported having greater positive feelings, clear-headedness, and fewer physical complaints. In addition, *the women reported fewer symptoms of PMS.*

Hormonal shifts can affect behavior and feelings, and they can be identified and managed better than we have done to date.[3] One thing women need to know is that there *are* physical imbalances, and they need to look at how they manage their stress, and what they are putting into their bodies that may further aggravate these imbalances. When the estrogen and progesterone levels are low, the blood sugar, serotonin, and endorphin levels are low, and the calcium/magnesium and salt/potassium levels are out of balance. *Sugar, alcohol, caffeine,* and *salt* may all drive these chemicals more out of balance.[4] So if you're taking these substances before your period, you may intensify symptoms of PMS.

Sugar, alcohol, and caffeine stimulate the pancreas to produce more insulin, and when this happens the blood sugar gets lower. Low blood sugar makes us feel emotional. We can feel too sensitive, and overreact to situations. Pre-menstrual women do report more accidents, and an inability to concentrate. Some are depressed and even suicidal. You may be intensifying these symptoms with the chemicals you put in your body.

Low progesterone causes low blood sugar, which can make some women crave sugar. Many pre-menstrual women crave chocolate which has sugar, caffeine, and magnesium in it, suggesting the body's yearning to correct the imbalances. The body tricks us, and unfortunately sugar (or alcohol, or caffeine) causes the blood sugar to go even lower, so if you take these things, you're in worse shape than when you started.

The foods that alleviate symptoms are complex carbohydrates, like whole grain breads and cereals, and green leafy vegetables—natural foods which elevate serotonin.[5] You can maintain balance within your system on a regular basis by eating protein every two or three hours. When you do this, insulin will not be overproduced and this avoids precipitously low blood sugar. The complex carbohydrates are considerably important any time from mid-cycle on, not only with respect to blood sugar but also as they relate to serotonin levels. The hormone drop causes serotonin levels to dip below what is comfortable for most women (serotonin is a brain chemical involved in sleep), and complex carbohydrates can help to steady that level. If PMS was the subject of rigorous investigation of the effects of hormonal fluctuation on behavior and mood swings, as often as it is the butt of jokes, we would have sufficient information on how to prevent mood swings.

Another result of low progesterone is that sodium is low pre-menstrually, causing the body to crave salt. If you eat salt, you may experience fluid retention. This can occur both in the abdomen and the brain. Minor fluid retention on the brain can cause sharp mood swings and make it difficult to think clearly. It helps enormously to avoid salt and salt-containing foods pre-menstrually (which means pretzels, ham, bacon, pickles, and yes—potato chips).

A great many of us do not take the time to eat properly. We may drink coffee and eat a donut for breakfast, and then go a long time before lunch, whereas eating a piece of fruit every couple of hours will keep the blood sugar level balanced and consistent. Proteins found in tofu, nuts, and yogurt also contribute to balance. We don't realize how much food affects how we think and feel. If you look at what you eat when you are very emotional, you can see how you actually *create* your own mood swings and feelings, as a result of what you swallow. We are creatures of habit, and in our culture we are taught from infancy to use food to comfort us. Consider for a moment the kind of thinking that wafts around us like smoke in a nightclub, the sensuous glorification of a "rich roasted" cup of coffee, gold-leaf chocolatiers, and sexy "soft" drinks (soft on who?—not on our blood system, our stomach lining, our cells, or our teeth, that's for sure).

Bad habits can be cracked wide open if we take responsibility for our own bodies. We can pledge to ourselves that "I am going to take control here, I am in charge, I am not a victim."

Some self-discipline is required. In Western health care, we are immoderately accustomed to popping into the doctor's office, getting a pill, and feeling better. If you are determined to feel better during PMS, a self-modulated care plan is necessary. *It does not come in pill form.* No manner of consistent good health does.

What to do?

Vitamin B complex tablets of 100 or 200 mg. daily, or 300 mg. daily just prior to the onset of PMS, can turn the tide of rising symptoms. Primrose oil, borage oil, or black currant oil capsules have been found by many women to be helpful because they produce linoleic acid, which is involved in the body's own generation of progesterone.[6] Primrose oil, Vitamin B, and complex carbohydrates are steps in the right direction. (Icing-laden cake, cookies, and ice cream are not.) Prepackaged PMS teas, or dandelion root, can relieve fluid retention. Valerian root tea or capsules can have a calming effect. Pro-Gest Cream, manufactured from wild yams, can also alleviate symptoms when rubbed on the soft tissue of the body (stomach or underside of forearms). Natural progesterone, taken in pill or suppository form prior to or during PMS, can be used if the other aforementioned holistic methods prove insufficient. Natural progesterone, available from the Women's International Pharmacy in Wisconsin, must be prescribed by your practitioner.[7]

Endorphins are low pre-menstrually, but if you exercise, endorphins are released, serotonin is increased, and both of these reactions can elevate your mood. Thirty to forty-five minutes of aerobic exercise, which releases anxiety and promotes tranquility, will counteract many symptoms by stimulating chemical changes within the body. Meditation relieves PMS symptoms by calming brain waves. Acupuncture has been used successfully to achieve balance and prevent PMS symptoms.[8]

Most importantly, it would be wonderful if partners could understand and acknowledge that PMS is a temporary hormonal imbalance, and support their partners in the implementation of these self-care measures. Thinly veiled ridicule has never been known to alleviate symptoms.

The holistic approach works wonders with PMS. In acute cases, I have given patients natural progesterone supplements in injections, pills, or suppository form. The results have been more successful when the women employ the holistic approach along with the progesterone. Artificial hormones (like birth control pills) can worsen symptoms of PMS. Start taking Vitamin B and primrose oil when you think you are getting PMS symptoms, and be aware of the food you are eating. It does take some effort, but once you add these ingredients to your daily recipe, they become routine. Nobody is a saint, but if you can remodel your diet a bit you will feel a lot better.

Some women report to me that when they have sugar premenstrually, they cannot work on a computer because they cannot concentrate or keep their fingers from shaking. Women have told me they become impatient with their children. One thing I stress to women is that if you know you're having PMS, don't schedule any stressful work or confrontations if it is at all possible. While at home, avoid corrosive arguments. Maybe you can say to your husband, "I need to go out for a walk, or to the gym. Could you watch the kids for an hour?" Do this when you know your alternative responses may be inappropriate.

It's great to know that you really can feel wonderful and re-born, and there is help out there and it works. You can do this yourself—change your diet and bad habits—and save money on medical visits and unnecessary tests.

Still, I don't think women can blame everything on PMS, or on hormonal imbalances. We have to look at our life, our lifestyle, and our relationships, and be honest about what is really going on. We need to differentiate between what is physical and what may be chemical imbalances—from food, drugs, or alcohol. We also need to consider the weight of stresses from jobs or families, because we are *whole* units. That is why my practice is called a "holistic" practice, and why I address each person as a whole unit—the mind, body, and the soul—wherein everything is connected. To think that an adolescent child calling from jail won't affect our physical health, for example, is a bit of folly. The way we handle the stress in our lives definitely impacts upon our health. By the same token, to think that eating the right food won't help is also folly.

During the second half of the menstrual cycle, after ovulation has occurred, our estrogen and progesterone levels are relatively low. This is called the luteal phase. ("Luteal" is a technical term used to describe changes that occur in the ovary after it discharges a mature egg.) Northrup has described this as the dark phase. She encourages us to go within ourselves during this time of month and listen to any messages our bodies might be trying to send us. If we can use this as a quiet, reflective time, we may find genuine truths about our lives, or answers to nagging questions. When women are in this phase of their cycle, they will often tell me they feel intolerant of their job or relationship, and that they wish they could work at something they love, or that fulfills their creative drives. I encourage them to pay attention to their own inner truth, and to make changes as they feel ready. In some cultures, women isolate together with other women before their menses, and in some Native America traditions they go into sweat lodges, because the menstruation is considered a sacred time for reflection.[9]

The holistic approach is almost nowhere more demonstrable than in reference to PMS, particularly as it relates to the "all in your head" brouhaha. My philosophy is that we cannot—either women or men—become victims of the health care system as it currently exists. Women traditionally have been heard saying, "Yes, doctor, I'll do whatever you tell me," whether it's take a pill, submit to surgery, or walk away believing you must be crazy because, after all, it's all in your head. I think there are other ways to look at health care, and other ways to maintain balance in your life. I'm not going to say "new" ways, because in many cases the methods I'm discussing have been around for thousands of years. For some reason, with the advent of the industrialized, computerized, laserized world, valuable old eating and exercise habits were lost or thrown out. To some degree, people simply lack information about this. If women were better informed about eating, exercise, stress management, and nutrition, *at any time of the month,* they could maintain better health. It's all about listening to your body and taking better care of it.

—8—

Perimenopause
and Menopause

Perimenopause, a period of months or years before meno-pause, can begin in a woman's mid-thirties and continue into the late forties or early fifties. When a woman has no periods for one full year, then she is menopausal. The average age at which menopause occurs is 50.4 years. These parameters are not rigid in a chronological or biological sense, but are subject to a wide range of human variation. "Peri" means "near" or "around," and so perimenopause refers to the time before menopause, which can last for up to 15 years. Perimenopausal women, who still have periods and are therefore not techni-cally menopausal, repeatedly come into my office talking about similar symptoms.

Common Complaints

One thing I hear over and over is that women report symptoms to their practitioners and ask if they are menopausal. The typical reply is, "No, you're too young." Their symptoms are worrisome although not life-threatening. I paid rapt attention to this issue when, at the age of 47, I got a speeding ticket and cried like a baby over it, and then later I felt I had grossly overreacted. My emotions sailed from one end of the spectrum to the other. Women at this age had told me they felt overemotional, or that they overreacted. They felt impatient with their children, or in-tolerant of things that used to be easy to manage, and naturally wondered, could this be menopause? When I explained to them it could be *perimenopause,* they felt relieved and validated. At least there was an explanation.

Another common symptom is memory loss. Women report they forget what they are saying in mid-sentence. There is a technical reason for this: estradiol levels are dipping. (Estradiol is the medical term for estrogen.) Throughout our lives we produce varying amounts of estrogen, which fluctuate throughout the day, as well as over the years. It's not a cause for alarm, but a fact to recognize and address with humor. Next time you forget what you are saying, just interject, "There goes my estradiol dipping again." Another side effect of estradiol dips is awakening in the middle of the night and not being able to get back to sleep.

The most common complaint concerns those infamous hot flashes that pop out of nowhere. Hot flashes occur during perimenopause as well as during menopause. A woman will feel hot all over, or her face will flush unexpectedly, or she will turn beet red or sweat profusely without warning. (I have a button that says these are "power surges, not hot flashes." It's essential to maintain our sense of humor.)

Women become anxious about these symptoms. When they are told it's not menopause, they think there must be something seriously wrong. Symptoms that could be addressed in a calm manner balloon into monstrous fears. For example, what happens in the case of hot flashes is simple. The ovaries produce less estrogen, which signals the hypothalamus (in the brain) to stop regulating heat production. It's as if a thermostat in your house stopped working and you could no longer regulate heat.

Irregular or rapid heartbeat can accompany hot flashes. Women often report feeling as if they are having a heart attack, when in fact it's normal hormonal changes. When the body loses estrogen, it is more prone to sympathetic nervous responses, so a typically perimenopausal loss of estrogen can trigger a stress response. Sympathetic nervous responses include rapid heartbeat, hot flashes, nausea, feeling faint, and emotional swings, all of which can occur during perimenopause. We can lessen these responses by avoiding caffeine, sugar, and alcohol, since they stimulate sympathetic nervous responses. When I am feeling emotional or having hot flashes, I try to remember whether I recently had sugar or caffeine.

Bladder problems such as frequent urination, burning, getting up at night, and incontinence, can also be symptoms of perimenopause. These occur due to loss of elasticity in the pubic coccygeal muscle, which is weakened by estrogen loss. This muscle surrounds the vagina and supports the bladder and rectum. It can lose elasticity following lack of exercise, childbirth, and/or lowering estrogen, causing loss of bladder and bowel control. Since the symptoms of urinary tract infections (UTIs) can be the same, it's important to be checked to see if infection is developing.

Skin, hair, and nails can become dry, and hair loss occurs also. Women are constantly asking me if hair loss and cracking nails are symptoms of menopause, and they can be.

Irregular menses can occur, ranging from experiencing no periods, skipping periods, having periods every two weeks, or constant bleeding. Periods can get lighter or heavier, more or less frequent. This is particularly unsettling if you are active physically and/or sexually. Fear of something serious, such as endometrial or ovarian cancer can arise. The genesis of irregularities is most often the lessening of estrogen and progesterone (another hormone). A complication is that ovulation can still occur, pregnancy can be a possibility, and irregular bleeding can be a sign of pregnancy. Thus the various signs, symptoms, and possibilities confuse us.

Loss of sexual drive is another concern. Women will tell me they just don't feel turned on, or that they have totally lost interest in sex. They wonder if this is part of menopause, and whether this means the end of their sex life. When I first began hearing this from perimenopausal-aged women, I turned to medical journals for some enlightenment, but in vain—there was little relevant. However, too many women were telling similar stories for it not to be considered typical. (Five hundred dissatisfied customers can't be wrong.) Dr. Philip Sarel, a psychiatrist at Yale University, who studies changes in the bodies of menopausal women, contends that lessening estrogen could contribute to a lowered sexual drive, but sex drive can be increased by taking Hormone Replacement Therapy (HRT).[1] Conversely, some women actually report an increase in sexual drive. This can happen as a result of decreased responsibilities as mothers and caretakers, freedom from worries about pregnancy, or the end of an unfulfilling relationship or marriage. As with everything, nothing is cut and dried or due to just one factor. Symptom origin is always multifactorial.

Breast tenderness, or the feeling of being pregnant premenstrually, is another common concern of perimenopausal women. The shift in balance between estrogen and progesterone causes breast discomfort. Of course, pregnancy is still a possibility at this time because you're still menstruating and, therefore, you can still ovulate even though it may happen irregularly. Women need to understand that breast tenderness could be a sign of pregnancy. Birth control methods are still necessary for sexually active women until there has been no period for one full year. This is hard to believe when you've had no period for seven or eight months, but it is a fact.

Perimenopausal women sometimes feel aching in their joints, shoulders, neck, and legs. Such aches resemble the symptoms of Lyme's Disease, and women sometimes think this is what they've contracted. (Lyme's results from a deer tick bite, but not from hormonal fluctuation.) However, osteoarthritis and osteoporosis can accompany the aging process, and they may produce symptoms at this time.[2] It does merit being differentiated from other potential diagnoses such as arthritis, Lyme's, Chronic Fatigue Syndrome (CFS), or Epstein Barr Virus.

In addition to a woman's estrogen and progesterone decreasing, sometimes her testosterone, which is the "male hormone" both sexes have, may fluctuate. Increasing testosterone levels may cause women to feel an increased sexual drive, while low testosterone decreases sex drive. (Dehydroepiandrosterone, or DHEA, another hormone contributing to sexuality, may also lower and result in decreased sexual drive.[3]) Women may suddenly have more facial hair, or they may notice that their voices deepen; this suggests increased testosterone. One woman told me she knew she was perimenopausal when she was tweezing more hairs from her lip than her eyebrows. These changes need not cause anxiety, and won't if women understand they are normal.

Serious Risks of Menopause

These perimenopausal symptoms range from being merely annoying to mildly painful. However, two potentially serious risks *may* develop once periods stop and menopause begins: osteo-porosis and cardiovascular disease. Osteoporosis develops when bones become extremely brittle due to calcium loss. At about age 30, women begin to lose bone mass, of which calcium is a chief component. This is a time when most women are drinking less milk or none at all, and incorporating less calcium into their diets in general. This alone can lead to loss of bone mass. Osteo-porosis can also develop from loss of estrogen and progesterone. In general, the thin, white, sedentary, smoking female is more prone to osteoporosis than others, and women who drink lots of caffeine, which robs the bones of calcium, are also more at risk.

Women can check for osteoporosis simply by measuring the span between each index finger with arms outstretched. If this measurement is less than your height, there may be some os-teoporosis developing. Osteoporosis can also be measured with a radiological scanning technique called Dual Energy Bone Densitometry (DEXA), which offers both accuracy and mini-mal radiation exposure. We women continuously lose some bone mass as we age, and we gradually become nine times more prone to bone fracture than men. Hunched-backed elderly women, slumped over due to shortening of their actual height, are the most obvious examples of osteoporosis. Hip, leg, and ra-dial (wrist) fractures are more common among menopausal women, all because of osteoporosis. As we will see, there are numerous holistic as well as conventional approaches to allevi-ating osteoporosis symptoms.[4]

Menopause can be coupled with cardiovascular risk. Tradi-tionally, we thought men were the primary candidates for heart attack; however, we are now finding some women are also at risk. Menopausal loss of estrogen increases risk for some women. As estrogen decreases, cholesterol that is usually transported away from the liver, in younger women, no longer leaves the older woman's system the way it once did. Instead, it slowly begins to line the blood vessels and can cause atherosclerosis, a thickening of the vessels from plaque (cholesterol deposits). Because of narrowed vessels, women can develop high blood pressure or even heart attacks, as less blood can flow to the heart.

Atherosclerosis develops when cholesterol adheres to and thus damages the walls of the arteries. Many factors contribute to this process including diet, stress, smoking, and lack of exercise. There are two types of cholesterol in the bloodstream. One type is called HDL, short for High-Density Lipoproteins. HDL is referred to as the "good" cholesterol because it clears out the arteries for smooth circulation. The other type of cholesterol is LDL, or Low-Density Lipoproteins. LDL is the "bad" cholesterol because it sticks to the arterial walls and cannot be cleared out by the body's usual methods. People have often looked at their cholesterol level (the combined total level of HDL and LDL) as an indication of cardiovascular health; however, we now know that cholesterol level does not tell the whole story. You can have a high cholesterol level and not be at risk for heart disease, because what is important is the relationship of LDL and HDL to each other—not their combined total level. The more good HDL you have, and the less bad LDL you have, the better—and this is true even if the *total* cholesterol level seems high. To figure out your HDL/LDL ratio, divide your total cholesterol level by your HDL level. A person with a ratio of 4.5 or higher (e.g., a total cholesterol of 225 divided by HDL of 50) is twice as likely to have heart disease as a person whose ratio is 3.5 (225 divided by HDL of 64). Obviously, these two ratios are different even though the total cholesterol level, 225, is the same. For many years, cholesterol levels hovering around 220 would have been considered dangerous. However, if your total is 220 and your HDL is 55, your HDL/LDL ratio will be 4.0, which indicates generally *good* cardiovascular health. The more "good" HDL you have, the better your circulation. The less HDL you have, the more problematic circulation becomes. In general, if your ratio is below 4.0, you are not at great risk for heart trouble. Measuring total cholesterol is meaningless without measuring the two separate types of cholesterol whose ratio to each other determines the risk factor for heart disease.[5] Many people with low cholesterol levels have had heart attacks, because their HDL levels were low.[6]

Not all menopausal women are at risk, but evaluations of the HDL/LDL ratio should be done at regular intervals once menopause begins. I agree with Betty Friedan, who in her book *Fountain of Age* cautions us not to buy into the medical myth that menopause is a disease and therefore all women are at risk for osteoporosis and heart trouble.[7] Risk is a highly individual matter, dependent upon both genetics and lifestyle, and must be separately assessed in every case. Generalizations do not apply here.

Holistic Approaches

A primary step for women is to take a look at what they eat.[8] As aforementioned, caffeine, sugar, and alcohol render women much more prone to disruptive sympathetic nervous responses. Caffeine in particular will induce these responses so rife with feelings of anxiety and emotionalism. Caffeine, sugar, and alcohol all lower the blood sugar level, and this can lead to hypoglycemia, which causes mood swings. As we lose estrogen and become more prone to sympathetic nervous responses, these substances will even more readily induce them. A vicious cycle ensues, leading to an even greater probability of a stress response. An estradiol dip can cause us to feel faint, or to overdramatize a speeding ticket, so we eat chocolate and have a cup of coffee and feel better. The physical combination of lowered estrogen plus coffee plus chocolate causes us to feel even hotter or more emotional, and the cycle starts again. This is when we need to start listening to our bodies. To chemicals that your younger self was able to put away, your body now says, "No, you cannot do that anymore, because you start having symptoms." Our bodies know they are losing estrogen; this is what is referred to as "the wisdom of the body." Admittedly, refusing coffee, or other like substances, may mean a change in routine for those of us who have spent our working lives with a cup of coffee—or many, many cups of coffee—at our desks at all times.

Eating sugar and drinking caffeine exacerbates emotional swings. When I was in the process of separation from a long-term relationship, I didn't know whether to attribute my frayed temperament to the separation, the caffeine, or the sugar. I was 47 at the time and perimenopausal. When I stopped consuming coffee and sugar, I had headaches and diarrhea for about two weeks, but I gradually began to feel more stable. Most importantly, I was able to sort out the disparate threads of my life and see what was due to caffeine and sugar, and what were the stressors associated with my relationship. Around this time I had a few car accidents, and I believe I was overwrought because of all the chemicals I had been putting into my body (*yes, caffeine and sugar are chemicals*). Like many of us, I thought these things would make me feel better, but the truth is they created even more stress. Loss of estrogen makes it difficult to metabolize these chemicals. A big cup of coffee with sugar can potentially cause a stress response in a 20-year-old woman, but her system is not at the mercy of fluctuating estrogen levels. So the actual physiological effect in a menopausal woman will be more disruptive than in someone younger. This is why we find ourselves wondering, "Why did this never bother me before? Why now?"

Hot flashes and racing heart rates are sometimes decreased by taking 600 to 800 I.U. of Vitamin E daily, 3000 mg. of Vitamin C, and 50 to 100 mg. of Vitamin B each day.[9] Vitamin B is particularly effective for stress, since stress literally drains our bodies of it. The combination of B, E, and C vitamins has been found to reduce hot flashes.

Perimenopause and menopause can make you feel overheated, so drinking lots of fluids helps. You wouldn't let your automobile engine overheat with no water in it, and it's the same with your body. Hydrating your body by flushing fluids through it decreases personal overheatedness. You can wear loose, cotton clothing that does not absorb and reflect heat. Sleeping with light cotton covers is helpful, although this may be difficult in a relationship when your partner is not having hot flashes, and you're throwing the covers off and he or she is pulling them back on! We need to reach some sort of compromise in relationships, and a sense of humor helps immensely. (Maybe this is why old movies featured couples in separate beds.)

Hot flashes can disrupt a deep sleep because estradiol tends to dip drastically at night. That's why it is so difficult to get back to sleep. It's important not to have caffeine, sugar, or alcohol before bed to help quell this midnight hubbub. If you take herbs or hormones to alleviate flashes and sleeplessness, they should be taken before retiring. In her book *Menopausal Years*, Susun Weed describes a cornucopia of useful plants and herbal antidotes to symptoms of menopause.[10] Weed's response to hot flashes might be to simply take a walk in the woods or the garden, and find a few good plants to eat.

Many people believe that some herbs lessen symptoms because they stimulate the adrenal glands—which sit over the kidneys—to produce more estrogen. If you're flushing your kidneys with water, that stimulates the adrenal glands, and herbs may do the same. Herbs commonly available in health food stores include dong quai, black licorice, sarsaparilla, black cohosh, ginger, or ginseng. There are combination preparations, specifically for menopause, on the market now, which are a mixture of these herbs together, and you can ask for them in most health food stores. They can be purchased in liquid or tablet form, or as teas. To combat the effects of decreased progesterone, primrose oil, black currant oil, or borage oil capsules made of linoleic acid are all helpful. Linoleic acid increases the production of progesterone. The herbs, oils and homeopathic preparations can be combined and used together, and may help in reducing symptoms.[11]

Stress reduction techniques such as meditation, yoga, massage, and acupuncture are antidotes to hot flashes. Acupuncture is particularly helpful because the kidney meridian can be stimulated to help the adrenal glands produce more estrogen.[12] Also, acupuncture can create balance in the body pathways—or meridians, as they are called in Chinese medicine. Balance attainment counters the feeling many women report of being "out of balance." Counseling, as a stress reduction technique, can be helpful because if stress is not handled effectively and continuously stimulates the adrenal glands, they will not function well.

To deter skin, hair, and nail dryness, keep the skin lubricated. Again, that means drinking many liquids, and lubricating your skin after bathing, when the skin will soak up oils like a sponge. A natural oil *with no alcohol or perfume* is the best choice. Olive oil is effective (Marilyn Monroe used it, so why not us?), as are sesame oil, corn oil, any type of vegetable oil, or Vitamin E oil. These are inexpensive ways to deal with skin dryness. When the body absorbs olive or safflower oil, the HDL/LDL ratio is improved, and this decreases cardiovascular troubles. It's also helpful to get some oil by mouth on a daily basis. This could be polyunsaturated oil such as vegetable oil, or mono-saturated types, such as olive oil. Our bodies need oil from the inside out as well as on the external skin.

Estrogen reduction can make women prone to vaginal infections, which can be avoided by staying away from sugar and alcohol.[13] Decreasing cheese consumption helps, too, as cheese can increase the chance of yeast infections. Women should not douche unless they really need to, because douching generally dries out the delicate vaginal tissues, and this renders them even more vulnerable to vaginal infection.

Vaginal dryness is a common complaint among sexually active menopausal women. Relief comes from keeping vaginal tissue lubricated on a daily basis, and I suggest that women put natural oil into their vagina every day. You can insert olive, sesame or safflower oil, or Progest Creme (made from wild yams, a natural form of progesterone) to combat dryness. You can put the oil on your finger and insert it into the vagina so that tissue remains lubricated. You can also insert a natural oil capsule into the vagina. Natural oils come in Vitamin E capsules, or Cod Liver Oil capsules, and they dissolve quickly. Just hold your finger inside for a few seconds until the capsule starts to dissolve, and this will naturally lubricate the tissue. Remaining sexually active, either by masturbating or with a partner, is an effective treatment because sexual activity stimulates lubrication. It's a case of "use it or lose it." Pharmaceutically available jellies and lubricants are helpful, although it is essential to use a water soluble jelly that does not dry out delicate tissues. Both you and your partner can utilize oils or jellies. Dryness should be discussed openly and honestly with a partner before a simple issue becomes a crisis.

Couples need to recognize that sexual and orgasmic responses may be slower at this time. If it takes longer to become lubricated, well, patience is a virtue. Couples can turn this into an asset, insofar as lovemaking can become slow and more relaxed than it was in the good old days. *Communication is of the essence.* If you are in a relationship with a man, he needs to know that if it hurts when he enters you, it's because of vaginal dryness. He needs to know that simply slowing down and using lubrication may help a lot. Many men are not aware of this, sometimes because women are afraid to talk about it. Men start to think they have hurt their partners, they lose their erection, then they think they're impotent, and then the woman thinks she is undesirable to her partner. And the next thing you know, nobody's having sex because both partners think they can't or they're unwanted and by this time they're both so full of resentment that who could make love anyway? All for lack of information! In the case of lesbian couples, both partners need to be aware of these facts with regard to insertion of objects into the vagina, how to deal with vaginal dryness, and changing sexual responses.

Menopause does not mean that sex life ends. It only means it has to change, and possibly slow down. Relax, enjoy, and *keep talking about it!* We need not think we cannot be sexual as we get older. People can maintain their sexuality for as long as they like, and that's because 95% of it is in the head. We need not buy into the myth that once you become older you cannot have sex. We need to keep talking about this openly and to set some new attitudinal precedents. I know many women who are sexually active into their sixties and seventies. They have been able to work through some of the discomforts of menopause to have an enjoyable sex life after menopause. It's not the same style they had as young women, but it's good just the same.

With respect to osteoporosis, preventive actions would include eschewing alcohol and smoking, and limiting intake of caffeine. These substances inhibit the body's absorption of calcium, and the body will rob the bones to make up for calcium deficit. Furthermore, a woman uses calcium less efficiently after estrogen production slows down, so it behooves us to increase calcium intake to 1500 mg. daily, with 750 mg. of magnesium also. (Women need 1000 mg. of calcium and 500 mg. of magnesium daily prior to menopause.) Calcium should be chelated since this is most easily absorbed by the body. "Tums" brand capsules are not a balanced source of calcium, although I know some medical personnel who prescribe Tums for women. Tums can actually upset the acid-base balance if taken in too large a quantity. It's better to obtain calcium from a vitamin capsule or from natural foods. Studies are now also showing the need for Vitamin D to help in the absorption of calcium (400–1200 mg. daily).[14] Pro-Gest Cream may also reduce osteoporosis.

Food can be used as medicine during menopause. For example, heaping a teaspoon of nonfat dried milk powder over breakfast or lunch, drinking calcium-fortified orange juice, eating one serving of low-fat yogurt, plus a dark green leafy vegetable, plus a one-inch cube of cheese each day will add about 1000 mg. of calcium to an ordinary diet. Combination vitamin capsules of Vitamin D, calcium, and magnesium are widely available (D and magnesium are necessary to absorb calcium). Apricots, nuts, broccoli, and sardines are good sources of calcium as well.

There has been recent concern within the medical community that when women do not have a natural source of estrogen, they cannot absorb calcium from pills or food.[15] Here "natural" means biological rather than externally introduced. Experts are not certain at this point, but I believe it is beneficial to consume calcium, magnesium, and Vitamin D in addition to herbs or hormone replacements.

Weight-bearing activity is an enduring weapon against the onslaught of osteoporosis. This includes activities such as aerobics, brisk walking, biking, roller blading, skiing, dancing, use of exercise machines, or any activity wherein you put weight on the long bones. It's helpful for menopausal women to exercise the bones of their wrists and forearms with light weight-lifting.[16]

Swimming, while beneficial in many areas of health, is not relevant to osteoporosis.

The combination of all these restorative efforts together—diets, herbs, exercise, and some prescription items—comprises a holistic approach to the alleviation of osteoporosis.

The holistic approach to reducing cardiovascular risk consists of aerobic activity on a regular basis. Aerobic means some form of activity where the heart is stimulated above its usual rate for 30 to 45 minutes, three to four times a week. These include all the exercises mentioned for osteoporosis. Walking is particularly effective, since it is not stressful on the joints, although we have to practice brisk walking in order to get the heart rate up. Again, it is crucial to maintain a low-fat diet, without any ice cream, whole milk, and minimal amounts of butter and meat. Avoiding animal fats should be your goal.

I monitor my menopause patients' coronary risk by drawing blood once a year to assess cholesterol level, triglyceride level, and HDL/LDL ratio. If cholesterol is above 200, the triglycerides are above 150, and the HDL/LDL ratio is above 5, the woman might be at risk for heart problems. The HDL needs to be high relative to the LDL, but LDL tends to increase and HDL decrease as estrogen goes down. Some women are thus at risk because a changing ratio means the liver is not transporting the fat away from the body. It is important to monitor this ratio as we age, because it indicates the need for medical attention. A good diet, herbs, and oils can help. For example, flaxseed oil has been shown to reverse the HDL/LDL ratio and keep it where it should be—yet another example of a naturally occurring substance doing what we often turn to prescriptions to do.[17]

Conventional Treatment and Controversies

If women find the natural oils don't work for them, prescription vaginal creams containing estrogen can be used for lubrication. They can be inserted into the vagina twice a week until lubrication returns, and then once a week or as needed after that. When used on a long-term basis, a woman needs to consider taking progesterone also, because the use of estrogen alone, in any form, increases the risk of uterine cancer. Premarin and Estrace Vaginal Creams are frequently prescribed estrogens. Natural estrogen cream made from soybeans is available from the Women's International Pharmacy Company.[18] Like synthetic estrogen, it is obtainable only by prescription.

Many women pass through menopause with no problems at all. Many experience discomfort, but not so much that it disrupts their lives or routines. It is more of a nuisance than a serious problem. Much media attention has been directed at hormone replacement therapy (HRT) during menopause, *but the truth is, not all women need it.* Prevention can be just as important as treatment, and women practicing holistic measures sometimes don't feel the need for HRT at all.

There are many types of estrogen and progesterone replacement.[19] Some women prefer an estrogen "patch," applied to the skin like a nicotine patch, because it bypasses the liver in a technical sense. If there has been a history of alcoholism or liver problems, they feel safer using the patch. Some women report that taking Estrace by mouth is most effective. Dr. Sarel recommends Estrace because it is most like the estradiol that the body itself produces. Some women use Premarin, by mouth, because it just feels right.

Estrogen dosages are started low, and if a woman's body doesn't respond, the dose is increased. Hormone levels can be measured. We can measure estradiol or perform a maturation index on a Pap smear, which indicates how many superficial cells are available and whether the body is responding to hormone treatment. If there are no superficial cells, then the body is not absorbing the estrogen and the dose needs to be increased.

HRT has been at the heart of much controversy. When I began working with menopausal women ten years ago, estrogen alone was recommended for reducing osteoporosis. This made me uncomfortable because studies were suggesting that although estrogen reduced osteoporosis, it increased cancer of the uterus by 300%! This is because estrogen constantly stimulates the lining of the uterus, causing a proliferative (thickening) endometrium. This leaves women more vulnerable to endometrial hyperplasia, which is a pre-cancerous condition of the uterus, or to actual cancer of the uterus. The medical community began to scrutinize this issue and to reexamine hormone replacement. Were the two benefits, decreasing heart disease and osteoporosis, greater than the increased risk of uterine cancer?

Gradually, research revealed that adding a smaller component of progesterone to the estrogen lowered the risk of uterine cancer.[20] The progesterone sloughed off the lining of the uterus on a regular basis (as it normally does in younger, non-menopausal women), thus eliminating the possibility of excessive stimulation by estrogen. Soon it became common to prescribe estrogen and progesterone in combination. Premarin (estrogen) is often prescribed in the amount of .625 mg. daily or Estrace is often prescribed at 1 mg. daily, or the Estraderm or Climara patch is often perscribed at 0.05 mg. daily. In addition,

Provera (progesterone), is often prescribed at 5 mg. on days 1 through 10 of the cycle, or 2.5 mg. every day.

Research has also shown that although progesterone was decreasing the risk of cancer of the uterus, it could increase the risk of heart disease by changing the HDL/LDL ratio.[21] The probability is that both osteoporosis and heart disease are drastically decreased by the presence of estrogen, but cardiovascular problems might be increased by progesterone. This leaves menopausal women who choose to use HRT caught between a rock and a hard place, trying to assess which course of action might be the lesser of two evils, and a substantial amount of study and questioning about HRT has taken place in the last ten years.

Often a woman's family history will dictate her course of action. Breast cancer, gallbladder disease, liver problems, and blood clots are some of the risks linked to HRT. More and more studies indicate that there is not a risk of breast cancer with short term hormone replacement (15 years or less). Furthermore, while replacement might increase some risks, it reduces that of osteoporosis and heart disease. This is significant because of the statistics: more menopausal women die from heart attack than from breast cancer.[22] The benefits could outweigh the risks, but still, each woman must make her own decision about risk/benefit ratio based on her philosophy, medical and family history, and lab data assessing her potential risks.

Some gynecolo-oncologists believe breast cancer survivors can take hormone replacements, but survivors I have spoken to generally do not want the risk associated with artificial estrogen. Each woman has to look at her own individual circumstances. If you have a family history of breast cancer, if you are a breast cancer survivor, if you have fibroids of the uterus, or *most importantly,* if your intuition tells you "don't take hormones," you should listen to your inner self when trying to decide what to do. Estrogen therapy may reduce coronary disease risk by 50%, but may increase risk of breast cancer, so the dilemma remains. More research needs to be done, and again, women need to listen to themselves after collecting information.

As aforementioned, the Wisconsin-based Women's International Pharmacy manufactures natural estrogen and progesterone, as alternatives to synthetic hormones. These can be taken by mouth or used in creme form. They must be prescribed by a practitioner just like synthetic HRT. These products are made from soybeans and other natural plants. Their estrogen product, TriEst, is 10% estrone, 10% estradiol, and 80% estriol. Plain estriol is also available. Since they are made from soy, which is phytoestrogen, they may lessen the risk of breast cancer. If you take any natural estrogen, it's important to keep in mind that you are still putting extra estrogen into your system, even though it's naturally derived and not synthetic. It's still estrogen and the possible risks still merit consideration.

W.I.P.'s Progesterone Cream, partially derived from soybeans, ensures the biological conditions for the body's own production of progesterone. Applied directly onto the soft tissue of the stomach, face, or forearms twice daily, it can relieve menopausal symptoms for many. Used vaginally, it combats dryness. Progest Creme made by Klabin Company has been assessed in terms of its reduction of PMS symptoms, vaginal dryness, and osteoporosis. Dr. John Lee has experimentally demonstrated that it is progesterone, not estrogen, that reduces osteoporosis.[23] He proffers that estrogen should only be taken short term for hot flashes and vaginal dryness, and that Pro-Gest Cream should be taken continuously to prevent osteoporosis. Progest Cream is available from Klabin Company directly, in some health food stores, pharmacies, or in practitioners' offices.

Sometimes women must make decisions based upon what appears to be conflicting data, and/or less scientific evidence. For example, one study found that 80 year-old-women who had only taken estrogen for five to ten years at the time of menopause had the same bone density as women who had never taken estrogen. Since the average age of hip fracture is 80, researchers are now suggesting women wait until age 70 to start HRT.[24] So each woman must decide for herself what to do, and if she does not want to take HRT for the rest of her life, she should consider whether holistic approaches might be more effective.

Some patients tell me that once they start taking hormone replacements, they feel better. The "edge is off," they are no longer plagued by emotional swings, and they are better able to cope with stressful situations. Their sex drive is increased, their vaginal dryness is diminished, and they just plain feel better. As one woman said to me, "I feel like my old self."

Some women try the holistic approach first, using herbs and changing their diet. If that doesn't help, they move on to the conventional. Some women try the conventional first, and they might have side effects such as mood swings from progesterone, or bloating and weight gain from estrogen, and then they try a holistic approach or natural HRT. You can combine both the alternative and the conventional together (*combining* approaches is an "holistic" method), and use them both in conjunction with one another.

We need to keep in mind that many women do not feel the need for hormone replacement at all, even though attendant publicity has often made them feel afraid they will develop severe problems if they do not take HRT. We should also be aware of any new scientific studies about hormone replacement. There is no one answer in terms of holistic versus conventional approaches to menopause. Many women have no symptoms or problems; they do nothing and seem to feel fine. However, a woman may be gliding through menopause without symptoms and then confront the death of a beloved parent, or her husband's triple bypass, or the loss of a job. Stress responses and the fluctuating hormones suddenly become a problem.

Women in their mid-forties who come into my office seem to be either adaptive or maladaptive. Maladaptive women are depressed, drinking, overeating, sedentary, and fatalistic. They become entrenched in stagnant thinking. Adaptation means that we try to turn difficulties around, to get counseling, to take chances, and to obtain more information about what is happening to our bodies. It means not giving in to the process of menopause and aging by saying, "My life is over, that's it for me." Adaptive women change right before my eyes. They become more creative about relationships—romantic, professional, and with their children. They're becoming more free and assertive about what their needs are, and about how they would like to see things happen.

Having choices about health care is alien to most women. Throughout history, we have so often not had choices. Where we lived, who or whether we married, where or whether we worked, and our economic status were dictated by our class, clan, tribe, or social stratum. We stand at a point in history where choosing health care is now critical to life. Unaccustomed as we are, it is time to take the reins, and menopause is a good place to begin. My experience has been that women who do take the reins find their purpose and commitment in life and, taking better care of themselves, have fewer emotional and physical problems during menopause. When I stop to think about it, many internationally influential women were or are menopausal, including Indira Ghandi, Eleanor Roosevelt, Betty Friedan, and Gloria Steinem. This suggests to me that menopause can be a time of great creativity, when you let go of old stereotypes and ideas. Margaret Mead talks about "menopausal zest," a time when women can really get outside themselves and take huge risks.[25] It is more positive to consider menopause as a transition—like adolescence. As I say in my workshops, it can be the pause that refreshes.

—9—

"Wellness" Defined

It is astonishing what an effort it seems to be for many people to put their brains definitely and systematically to work. They seem to insist on somebody else doing their thinking for them.

Thomas Edison[1]

Suzanne takes sixteen different medications, and she doesn't know if she's coming or going. The doctor prescribing her pills does not know she's a recovering addict and alcoholic, because he has little time to talk to her. Addicts can become hooked on any pharmaceutical product, and Suzanne takes numerous pills. I asked her if any medical professional ever talked to her about taking care of herself, or accepting responsibility for her diet. Her answer, like many others, is "no."

When she comes into my office, I talk with her about taking care of herself. I don't know whether she's ready for this, because as much as we complain about the medical establishment, we still go to practitioners expecting to be told what to do, and to be given pills and medications. These expectations are something we ourselves create, and the medical establishment has traditionally obliged us. I no longer think this is what patients want.

Ingrained Attitudes: Teaching Old Dogs New Tricks

Attitudes about wellness get twisted into position, like wet ropes knotted together and dried steel-hard. Cultural shibboleths and ingrained axioms are hard to change, even when they make us sick. Illness results when we don't take care of ourselves, while "wellness," conversely, is all about *responsibility*. That responsibility is for our health, our well-being, and our bad habits.

Wellness refers to a lifestyle designed to prevent illness. Components of wellness include exercise, nutrition, avoidance of known environmental toxins, regular check-ups, a spiritual process, and *awareness* that these variables either promote or detract from wellness. A "wellness model" contradicts the "illness model" too often invoked by the medically dominant U.S. health care system. We health care professionals have often treated illness with pills and surgery, rather than explaining to people how to cooperate with their bodies to stay well. When we get sick, we should begin to think in terms of striving for balance, rather than for a quick pharmaceutical fix.

A friend of mine was asked by a gynecologist how she felt during PMS, and she replied that she felt "off the wall." He gave her a prescription for Prozac. It's a frightening fact of modern medicine that when people get emotional, or upset, or have PMS, they are given Librium, Valium, Prozac, or other like drugs. Then they get hooked and need more and more, and nobody's ever spoken to them about taking responsibility for their own wellness, how to take care of themselves, or what's going on in their lives. Is it physiologically incorrect to have PMS? Or have we convinced ourselves that it is?

Most of us do not think of ourselves as working toward staying well every day. We ignore the issue until we get sick, and then complain because we have pain. For example, we don't usually think of using food as medicine, although that approach has been integral to Chinese medicine and other ancient disciplines for thousands of years. If we did use food as medicine, we would begin to think of food differently. As it is, our cultural decrees make it socially acceptable to take chemically manufactured antacids for indigestion, but if we mention papaya or peppermint—natural aids to digestion—we are laughed out of the room. What's going on here? Why is the synthetic facsimile acceptable, while a natural remedy is comical? And more to the point, *why do we wait until we get really sick to think about this?*

The Multifactorial Nature of Wellness

In order to live a lifestyle designed to regain or maintain wellness, we must acknowledge that all illness is multifactorial. Illness is caused by many things, and never the result of one single factor. Wellness is also multifactorial. A holistic approach to health care means consideration of the *whole* person, and not just *some of her parts.* Owning up to what we ourselves must do means looking at our whole lifestyle, not just *some* of our habits. Getting adequate exercise but continuing to smoke won't necessarily result in wellness, because both factors—exercise *and* smoking—are involved in wellness. Eating nutritiously but getting no exercise, again, does not take into account all of the many factors of wellness. There's an old cliche—"all things considered"—and in the case of maintaining wellness, all things must be considered, not just the "thing" we want. Many of us like to exercise, but are nonetheless bedeviled by juicy steaks or Belgian chocolates. Overdoing one factor won't purge the skipping over of another.

Regular exercise is one of the multiple factors contributing to wellness. When we exercise, chemicals called "endorphins" are released from the brain, from the adrenal glands, the hypothalamus, the pituitary, and the thyroid. Exercise is a major part of the "mind-body connection." When I'm really agitated, or have something that I need to work out, if I go out and run, ride my bike, or do something physical, I feel better. The action of exercising somehow alters the stress level. Part of this has to do with the release of endorphins. Another part could be that my perception of myself improves when I exercise.

Exercise strengthens and tones the muscles, so they are more fit and working consistently. It increases metabolism, burns more fat, and gets rid of toxins. People on diets who don't exercise don't lose weight. Their metabolism just slows down. They develop a set weight at which their body is comfortable. If they decrease what they eat, the body notices and says to itself, "She's going to starve me, so I'm going to store up fat and just hang onto it. Then when starvation comes, I've got something to burn up." This is why so many dieters are frustrated. You have to both decrease food intake and simultaneously increase metabolism to lose weight.

As exercise speeds up metabolism, blood flow to every organ in the body increases. The brain, heart, liver, and kidneys all work more efficiently. Regular exercise leads to a slower heart rate, which means the heart is working more efficiently because it has to beat less frequently. Like an engine in a car, the less it has to work, the better. The more it has to work, the sooner it wears out.

Exercise improves immune system functioning by circulating toxins to move them out of the body via the liver and kidneys. The function of the liver is to detoxify, so if you're exercising and increasing the blood flow to the liver, you eliminate a greater amount of toxins. We all carry toxins, and the more efficiently the body works, the more efficiently we get rid of them. This may explain why some people get sick and others don't. Some people seem to be exposed to a lot of toxins, yet they never get sick.

If we are not exercising currently, half an hour a day every other day would be a good start, or half an hour to forty-five minutes, three to five times a week. You have to increase heart rate to produce any genuine or long-lasting results. There is cardiovascular benefit inherent in increased heart rate, because the heart muscle gets toned. Like any other muscle in the body, it works more efficiently when toned. Regular exercisers cope with stress more effectively because their hearts and adrenal glands are running smoothly. The adrenals are the glands primarily involved in stress, and in the case of a well-toned heart and adrenals, everything is being pumped through and out before it can settle in and cause trouble.

Risk factors for certain illnesses including heart attacks and strokes are decreased by regular exercise. Frequent exercise allows the blood to flow more freely, so vessels aren't clogged. A clot cannot stick to the wall when it's forced to keep moving. If we don't exercise, we could get high blood pressure, in part because the arteries become clogged with plaque. This makes the heart work extraordinarily hard, so the blood pressure soars. If it goes high enough, pressure is pitted against the artery wall all the time. Eventually the walls weaken and pop, and blood seeps out where it should not be.

Hypertension patients are often advised to get more exercise. You may think, "If I exercise my blood pressure will go up," but the long-term benefit of exercise is lowered blood pressure, due to improving the tone of the vessel walls.

Dr. Dean Ornish's work stands as a stunning and enduring testament to the power of exercise and other wellness factors.

His book, *Dr. Dean Ornish's Program For Reversing Heart Disease,* explains how diet, exercise, and relaxation techniques have saved the lives of numerous heart patients who sought his help.[2] The same can be said of the Pritikin Institute in Florida, where people facing open heart surgery are placed on a program of regular exercise, significant dietary changes, meditation, and classes in stress reduction techniques.[3] After incorporating this program into their lives, they often don't need surgery. Some people go to Pritikin *after* bypass surgery, so they can learn a preventive style of living to avoid further surgery.

During a bypass, the patient is hooked up to a heart and lung machine. All their blood is purified, and then recirculated into the body. Despite the complexity and danger of a bypass, many people seem to be intractable about coronary artery disease and surgery. They don't seem to grasp that, if they made some changes in their lives, they might not need surgery. This applies even to those who have survived the painful and difficult post-operative experience. Here are people who have been anesthetized for long periods of time, they've endured major invasion of the body, and they still don't understand that they need to make some changes, or their arteries will get clogged again.

One woman I saw had undergone three bypass surgeries. I don't know whether cases like hers are the fault of the medical community, in that practitioners don't tell patients what can be done and that habits must change, or whether some people just don't want to hear the truth. They don't want to make the tremendous effort toward lifestyle changes that prevent illness, surgery, or death.

When he was a conventional physician, Deepak Chopra told a patient that if he would stop smoking, eat differently, and exercise, he could get out of the intensive care unit. The patient replied that his mother-in-law had told him the same thing, but he didn't have to pay her.[4] That reply got Dr. Chopra thinking. Shortly thereafter, he began his study of Aruyvedic medicine, an ancient Indian study of the biochemical changes which result from lifestyle changes. Deepak Chopra has become well-known for his books and articles on these issues, and has founded a clinic in Delmar, California, to serve people with serious illnesses. Most of his clinic patients come from conventional medical settings where they tended to get worse instead of better. Chopra was a conventional American doctor, and he has combined that training with a decidedly non-traditional philosophy. Many of us who complete traditional medical or nursing training are not open or exposed to novel approaches to prevention and wellness. I never was. During my nursing training, my total exposure to nutrition consisted of learning about the diabetic diet. I began studying nutrition on my own because I believed there must be some connection between poor nutrition and disease, and between good nutrition and health. Working with patients made that very obvious to me. Nevertheless, we have a situation where not only are most patients resistant to change and new thinking, but so are many practitioners. Many of us, *on both sides of the fence,* are resistant to changing our thinking, our habits, and our health science and medical school curriculum.

If you're not well, ask yourself, "Am I exercising? How much do I exercise? What can I do to put this into my life?" It's important to do something you like. Some people like to take classes, or go biking with friends, while others prefer solitary walks and jogs. We each need to determine what works for us specifically.

The biggest problem for most women is finding the time. While an hour's exercise a day might be optimally desirable, we have careers, children, elderly parents, family illnesses, and other realities that make that kind of time slot laughable. This is where thinking of wellness as a priority, and changing our traditional thinking, enters in.

And speaking of traditional thinking, nowhere does it merit a good skewering than on the topic of nutrition. There are so many times when a patient seeks medical help and is given a prescription for a drug, when what he or she should have been advised to do was make an appointment with a nutritionist. When it comes to wellness and eating, many of us have never seen the two as connected. Consider how often the term "Mama's cooking" refers to both maternal affection and gravy followed by homemade pies. Gravy in this context means lard-laden, and pies are the kind with sugar. My grandmother, whom I adored, made lots of chocolate cake and fudge, and I got mired in her message too well. I recently ate a bag of chocolate chips because I was upset with someone. The next morning I felt awful. I spilled water all over my dress just before starting work, and I was disoriented because chocolate is loaded with sugar. For me, I knew I was stuffing my feelings, and not eating because I was hungry. We ought not use, *or misuse*, food to eradicate stress. Instead, food should be used as a healer. There are numerous stress reduction techniques we can embed into our routine, but overeating should not be one of them. Indeed, we need to be careful with food, because its misuse has a boomerang effect. We eat to feel good, but wind up with obesity and clogged arteries, which don't feel real good.

Some foods create illness. Food high in animal fat—as present in red meat, cheese, ice cream, and Mama's gravy—open up many questions. My paramount concern about red meat though, is this: what are the cows being fed? What kind of nutrition are the cows getting? What is injected into cows, in terms of hormones and other drugs, and into chickens, too? Currently, research suggests that some nutritionally devastating procedures are visited upon chicken products.[5] Chicken is unpalatable after you read some of this research. There are many things we don't know about what happens to the animals we eat.

Even when or if chickens are healthy, there is a good deal of fat in their skin. In some cases, it might be better to have shrimp or other shellfish rather than chicken, because although shrimp has cholesterol, it doesn't have animal fat. If you eat chicken, you should always consider removing the skin, or else you're getting just as much fat as red meat.

When I ask my patients how much fat they eat, they say they don't eat red meat at all. Still, they can't lose weight, they have high blood pressure, heart problems, soaring cholesterol levels, and their HDL/LDL ratio is not healthy. They're eating cheese every day, and they think cheese isn't fat. I don't know where people think cheese comes from, but it comes from animals' milk, and it is often a culprit in high fat diets.

If you reduce the amount of animal fats in your diet, you may prevent heart disease and stroke, as well as some cancers. Fat causes plaque to build up in the blood vessels, and soon the flow of blood to the heart is decreased. If there is not enough oxygen and blood flow to the heart muscle, heart attack occurs. Stroke takes place under similar conditions.

Fat is involved in many cancers. Among the Japanese, the incidence of bowel and breast cancer is very low. When Japanese immigrate to the U.S. and start to eat fat typical of the American diet, their incidence of heart disease, breast cancer, and bowel cancer climbs dramatically.[6] I believe there are other contributing factors, such as our stressful lifestyles, but certainly diet is a major factor. Illness—and wellness—are always multifactorial. The combined effects of diet, nutrition, exercise, work habits (manual and sedentary), and stress contribute to illness and wellness.

There are nine calories in a gram of fat, but only four in a gram of protein or carbohydrate. When you really crave a snack, it would be better to indulge in carbohydrates or protein. The body does not metabolize fat easily, but stores it in the muscles and tissues, which makes it almost impossible to burn up. This is not news to repeat dieters.

When it comes to foods that feed disease, sugar looms large, sometimes larger than life.[7] When we ingest sugar, the pancreas is forced to discharge a higher than normal level of insulin into the body. When the pancreas shoots out more insulin, our blood sugar level drops down, causing a hypoglycemic condition. Eventually the pancreas, driven to an unnatural level of overwork, capsizes in a sea of sugar, and the result is diabetes. Sugar is a slow, silent killer. If you leave a human tooth in a glass of cola (which is pure sugar) overnight, you will find the tooth eaten away the next morning. Furthermore, sugar-loving bacteria grow inside the body. In his book, *The Yeast Connection*,

Dr. William Crook explains how sugar ferments inside our bodies.[8] People who eat a lot of sugar—or beer, cheese, and wine, which also ferment inside the body—will have sugar settling into the bowel, where it ferments and grows. Eventually they get chronic yeast in their bowel, with the yeast backing up into the bloodstream and destroying the immune response. Dr. Crook developed his theories about the "yeast connection" after seeing many patients with allergies, sinusitis, and asthma. He found himself treating these allergies over and over in vain, so he set about trying to find out what caused them in the first place.

Crook put his patients on a yeast-free and sugar-free diet, and instructed them to take acidophilus every day. Acidophilus creates lactobacillus, and is the main ingredient in yogurt. The presence of lactobacillus suppresses bacteria. If you have enough lactobacillus in your system you basically won't grow yeast. Crooks's patients took acidophilus three times daily, either in liquid or tablet form, as well as caprylic acid or Nystatin, which kills yeast from the inside out, and this regimen cleared out their systems. They started to get better. I have suggested this regimen to many patients. (They take Nystatin if the caprylic acid doesn't work. Nystatin is a prescription item, and I always try the natural product first, which in this case is caprylic acid.) People have reported to me that symptoms have cleared up, including those of sinusitis, chronic yeast infections, irritable bowel syndrome, and fatigue. People start to feel better and they lose weight, because, of course, they're eating no sugar, and they're eating natural foods instead. In our culture, we have something of a mental logjam where sugar is concerned. We cannot seem to break through to where we see its danger clear-eyed. When an oversized cake is rolled out at a party, people tend to cheer, whereas the more appropriate response might be to recoil with healthy fear.

In addition to fat and sugar, some preservatives may be unhealthy. We don't know precisely what is in some food preservatives, and some are not natural products. The effects of pesticides, and numerous other external toxins are not yet fully understood either.

Alcohol is a self-applied toxin. It destroys the liver and the immune response, as do marijuana, heroin, and cocaine. These substances put the body through a blender. First it's up, then it's down, and the whole system—the adrenal glands, the pituitary, the thyroid—are really out of balance. If things are not in balance, the body is not going to work properly, and it is going to get sick. All disease is a symptom of something being out of balance.

Vegetables and fruits contribute to wellness because they contain vitamins and fiber. In other cultures throughout the world, people eat a great many fruits and vegetables because that's what they find around them. They do not have legions of prepared, packaged, oversweetened, oversalted, chemically processed, technologically wilted food from which to choose. The fiber in *raw* fruits and vegetables helps to eliminate toxins from the system so that everything keeps moving through the body, rather than becoming clogged. A high fiber diet can decrease the incidence of diverticulitis, an inflammation of the bowel. We are talking now about raw foods, not canned, frozen, or overcooked. Then, too, the best way to cook is by steaming and stir-frying quickly.

With respect to fats, there are certain fats we need. The "good" fats are found in fish and olive oil, both of which can actually lower cholesterol and the HDL/LDL ratio (see Chapter 8 for explanation of the HDL/LDL ratio). There is always cholesterol in the body and it comes in two types, high density lipo-protein (HDL) and low-density lipo-protein (LDL). Ideally, the HDL is high and the LDL is lower. If their ratio to each other is balanced like this, it means your liver is transporting the bad fats away from the blood vessels. If the ratio is reversed, with low HDL and high LDL, then your liver is not effectively flushing out the bad guys, and they tend to stick to the blood vessel walls. HDL transports fat away from the liver, keeping blood vessels open.

We all produce some degree of cholesterol naturally, no matter what we eat. Some people have a genetic pre-disposition to high cholesterol, but their levels can be lowered with medication. For most of us, however, cholesterol levels are a function of what we eat, whether we exercise, and what toxins worm their way into our bodies. The HDL/LDL ratio stays where it should be with low animal fats in the diet, regular exercise, giving stress an outlet, and lowering the amount of toxins (such as alcohol and cigarettes) that you allow into your body. As we discussed in Chapter 8, as menopausal women lose estrogen, they can become more prone to heart disease. Their HDL/LDL ratio veers off because lowering estrogen makes the body less able to transport bad fat away from the liver. Flaxseed oil capsules, as well as olive oil, can help keep the HDL/LDL ratio where it should be.[9] There are pharmaceutical medications you can take to address menopause and high cholesterol, but I always try the natural things first, *especially renovating the diet.*

If you are vegetarian, or a macro-biotic eater, you still need some type of protein. Beans and rice combined is a good protein source, as are low-fat cheeses and yogurt. Nuts, although they do contain vegetable fat, are good because they do not have animal fat. Again, as we discussed in previous chapters, blood sugar level remains constant if you eat protein every two to three hours. If you carry nuts and raisins to snack on every three hours or so, you cut your risk of becoming hypoglycemic. We need to come to grips with this truth: The food we put into our bodies alters our biochemistry. There is no way around, through, under, or over this, our blizzard of rationalizations notwithstanding.

The American Dietary Association recommends what is called the "Triangle" of carbohydrates, proteins, and fats. The bottom and largest part of the triangle is what you want the most of, 60% carbohydrates. Proteins should comprise 20% to 30%, as the middle of the diet triangle. The tip-top of the triangle, the last 10% to 20%, should be fats, and that is a balanced diet. Our diet in the past had fat at the bottom of the triangle and carbohydrates at the top. This literally creates illness, so when you go food shopping, look for fresh fruits and vegetables, brown rice, potatoes, pasta, and breads and cereals. Breads and cereals should be whole grain, as there is no nutrition in bleached white flour. And there's no nutrition in sugar. People mistakenly suppose sugar is a carbohydrate, but it's not. It is highly caloric but nutritionally empty. It will keep you going for a while, deceptively, but eventually you crash.

When we do not get enough vitamins naturally from the intake of food, vitamin supplements are needed. Depending upon individual preference, both water soluble and fat soluble vitamins are available. Water soluble vitamins are B and C, which are easily excluded, or excreted, from the system when not needed. When you take high-potency vitamins, you notice that your urine turns yellow. Some practitioners contend that taking vitamins is a waste of effort because they just get lost in the urine. Conversely, some patients on high doses of Vitamin C seem to recover from all manner of illness.

Vitamins do differ in their levels of toxicity. Neurological deficits have resulted from overdoses of Vitamin B, proving that supplementation is not an arena where if a little bit is good, a lot will be wonderful.

Vitamins A and E are fat soluble, which means they are stored in fat cells and are thus not as easily excreted. The body tends to hold onto them, and they can build up to toxic levels. Care must be taken when patients with acne take high doses of Vitamin A. It's splendidly healing to the skin, but not in toxic doses. Yellow vegetables such as carrots and squash are natural sources of Vitamin A. Vitamin E helps to maintain a sound HDL/LDL ratio, and it's also involved in decreasing PMS. Some researchers think it's a cancer preventive, and others believe it keeps the sex drive healthy.[10] There have been multitudes of theories expounded on what vitamins can and cannot do. Each of us, individually, needs to consider the myriad vitamin theories, separate the wheat from the chaff, and determine what we think is best for ourselves. The best sifter we have to strain vitamin therapies through is called "intuition."

Wellness maintenance means having lots of liquids in our diet, and the best one is water. Where pollution is a concern, I suggest bottled water. Basic, mundane old water is not only effective in flushing everything from the body, but it also prevents dehydration. The thinking parts of our brain don't work effectively when we are dehydrated. The bladder doesn't function, other organs will slow down, toxins will build up, and skin and hair will be dry.

Spirituality and Health

Each individual must find his or her own path to wellness, one that supports his or her belief system. Just because we adopt a few externally visible wellness techniques (like publicly eating brussels sprouts), we are not assured of optimal health, because internal, spiritual factors are also involved. When I think about healing, I think of the mind, body, and spirit as a trilogy; all three must be addressed to achieve wellness. You can come to an understanding of this by using whatever works for you personally, whether it's meditating, playing or listening to music, prayer, being at one with nature, creating art, writing, exercising or whatever means you have for accessing energy for wellness. Bernie Siegel, M.D., author of *Love, Medicine, and Miracles*, states that prayer can bring peace of mind, solace, and inner strength, all of which are powerful medicine.[11] By turning to a source within ourselves, one that we know works for us and brings us personal peace, we can deal with stress more effectively, stay in the parasympathetic nervous response, and elevate the immune response. My patients with life-threatening illnesses who have healed themselves list a spiritual process as a major component of the work they do. Often in Western medical offices, the spiritual path is ignored, but I find it to be an integral part of holistic health.

Joan Borysenko has written several books on PNI wherein she stresses the spiritual process as an important part of wellness.[12] For example, she points out how Alcoholics Anonymous is an integral tool for members to express their feelings, arrive at forgiveness, and let go of resentments, and she shows how this elevates the immune response. Personally, I have found I need a spiritual process to help me achieve optimal wellness, because it helps to break down the barriers between the mind and the body. In *The Spirituality of Imperfection,* authors Ernest Kurtz and Katherine Ketchum quote Alcoholics Anonymous founder Bill Wilson, who said, "We must find some spiritual basis of living, else we die."

Our bodies will always tell us how they feel in relation to exercise, food, and stress, so listen to yourself. Wellness is achieved through a variety of approaches, with no one road leading to Rome. The individual sense must emanate from your inner voice.

–10–

Self-Advocacy

In my position as Patient Advocate at a large, bustling hospital, I was accustomed to frantic calls, but this one seemed more urgent and anguished than usual. Two surgeons were requesting that I speak with a patient they were about to take into emergency surgery. I rushed to the floor not quite knowing what to expect. Mrs. Smith was sitting up in bed, surrounded by nurses and technicians. On her left leg was an ulcer the size of a melon—a stasis ulcer, which had developed as a result of poor circulation. Cleansing and saline compresses are the normal treatments, but Mrs. Smith had waited too long to seek help, so it was beyond such treatment.

"It's so badly infected that it has maggots in it!" one of the nurses explained. "We clean it out with Betadine and disinfect it every day, but it's so far gone it doesn't improve." I had never seen maggots in a hospital before, but I salvaged my composure.

"They want to amputate my leg," Mrs. Smith said to me. "But I won't let them."

"Mrs. Smith," began Dr. Wade, the chief of surgery, "if we don't amputate now, you are going to die."

"I don't care," she replied. "I don't want my leg amputated."

Dr. Wade took me aside. "Reason with her, please." I explained to him that if the patient did not want the amputation, we could not do it. "Make her understand that she is going to die without it," he told me, as he stormed away impatiently.

I asked everyone to leave so I could sit with Mrs. Smith quietly. I explained to her that she could almost certainly die if she did not agree to the amputation.

"I don't care," she said and looked out the window, not seeing the trees and the traffic, gazing past them to the time long ago and far away in her memory, grimacing in pain at wherever it was taking her. "My mother spent the last years of her life with both legs amputated, in a wheelchair, and I'm not going to live that way. It was a nightmare for her. And for me, too. I'd rather die than live that way."

"Are you sure you understand that you are going to die?" I tried one last time. She nodded. "It's my job to make sure you understand this." She understood.

I left to find the surgeons. I told them we could not operate without her permission, and she wasn't going to give it. They were furious. "You've worked as surgical nurse," one of them blared at me. "How can you allow this? What's the matter with you?" Intimidated and shaking, I repeated to them that it wasn't up to us. It was her decision, and she was competent and aware of what she was deciding. "This is ridiculous," Dr. Wade muttered as they all walked away angrily.

Every day for 21 days, Mrs. Smith's abscess was cleaned out with antiseptics by the nurses. Inexplicably, it began to heal. Now that I understand PNI, my belief is that the patient's determined attitude, coupled with careful nursing care—cleansing the wound to rid it of bad tissue so that good, healthy, new tissue could grow—allowed healing to occur.

On the twenty-eighth day, Mrs. Smith walked out of the hospital on her own two legs, completely cured of the ulcer that had threatened her life.

That experience stayed with me for many years, showering light on my thinking about the role of a fighting human spirit in physical health. My philosophy about the connection between spirit and health was never the same after that. My own outlook became more fluid, rather than static and immovable. Mrs.

Smith taught me that many factors, in addition to the obvious factors we professionals learn about in chemistry or anatomy class, contribute to healing. Years later, after I had become a nurse practitioner and opened my own women's health care practice, I thought of Mrs. Smith when another frantic phone call came in.

Anna, a patient of mine, was calling from a busy clinic that offered walk-in services for general medical complaints. Her ear had hurt for several days, and she had gone to the clinic with what she felt was an ear infection. The physician who saw her told her she needed a vaginal examination to determine whether a yeast infection was causing her ear pain.

"I just wanted to run this by you," Anna said on the phone. "Have you ever heard of doing a vaginal exam for ear pain?"

"It doesn't seem appropriate to me," I replied. "What are you going to do now?"

"Well," she started to cry, "I let him do a vaginal exam already."

"Why did you do that?" I asked, "when your intuition told you it didn't make sense?"

"I don't know," she cried, "but he didn't find any yeast infection." I cried with her. "He's the doctor, you know?" she whispered.

I told her to find the manager of the clinic immediately and explain what happened. She hung up the phone, found the chief administrator, and told him about the exam. The doctor was fired that day.

A misbehaving practitioner was weeded out because Anna chose to *listen to herself,* just as a leg was saved because Mrs. Smith *listened to herself.*

How can we begin to listen to ourselves, so that we do not loose our dignity and our choices?

If It's Broke, Fix It

There's an old saying, "If it ain't broke, don't fix it." If the way we interact with health care providers is not working for us, then the opposite is true. It *is* broke, and we *should* fix it. Just how will we undertake the task?

Women can become equal partners with their health care providers, *but not by magic.* We need to make arduous choices, choices we know are right for us, and *not* what might be right for everybody else, or what everybody tells us, or what society tells us. We need to be our own investigators, and we accomplish this by gathering an abundance of information from reading and talking to others. The way to "fix it" is to be our own advocates, and to achieve self-responsibility rather than accepting passivity.

The first and most important aspect lies not with the legal details of patients' rights, practitioners' mistakes, or hospitals' inefficiencies. Rather, it concerns what goes on deep inside our own heads: *thinking.* The first step we need to take is toward being flexible and conducive to changing our minds about the inevitability of the current system. If we can change our thinking about how health care is or should be delivered, then we can begin to take concrete steps toward taking better care of ourselves. However—and this is key—*we cannot wait until we are sick, tense with illness, and timid in the face of unknown fears.* Once we become ill, the fear factor wields too much influence.

Like wellness, self-advocacy should begin to reverberate through our lives long before we get sick, so that an open-minded philosophy is already in place, so to speak, when crisis strikes.

Simple vigilance and everyday alertness are adequate tools. One need not be a lawyer or learned professor to ask simple questions. For example, we have probably all heard about, or lived through, the habit some practitioners have of ordering unnecessary tests and therapy, sometimes at facilities they own. If we are suspicious about tests, we can report them to a local Medicaid Fraud Control Unit at the office of any state attorney general. The very focus of these offices is to investigate the ordering of excessive tests. We can also write to the National Association of Attorneys General, 444 N. Capitol Street, Suite 339, Washington, D.C. 20001, for information about how to pursue an investigation in states where there is no local Fraud Control Unit.

In some fashion, we have tacitly and unknowingly permitted ourselves to become victims of the health care system, and this is what needs fixing. How has it come to pass that we let medical practitioners tell us what to do with our bodies, accept what they tell us, and then, when we don't get better, blame them? It would be better to become *partners with our practitioners*, and if we are not made to feel like partners, then we can choose a different practitioner. In this way, we can begin to feel reliant upon and trusting of the system, rather than undone by it.

The current situation was designed or has evolved so that practitioners are, in one way or another, revered—revered perhaps less now than then, but still much too much. Practitioners are expected to look down at patients and somberly proclaim,

"I know more than you and you have to listen to me or you'll suffer, even die." In response, patients may start to stay away, they may not come for help. They may not ask questions and if they don't ask questions, they become victims who have no say. *If they have no say, they can rationalize taking no responsibility for being well.* That thrusts us into the role of having to know everything. I used to think I had to have all the answers, because people expected that of me. When I started giving them responsibility for themselves, they got worried. Now people come to me *because they know they will be challenged.* They will be asked to think about what they want in their health care, not what I think is right. I give them lots of information and they make their own choices.[1]

Cultural attitudes in many ways buttress the medical establishment. When I am with patients, I never use the word "patient" in our conversations together. In their presence, I tell them they are "clients." When people are directly addressed as "patients" it connotes that they are "sick," and I don't like people coming into my office thinking they are "sick." I prefer to have them think they have the potential for being well. What they have is an imbalance, and imbalances can be brought back into balance.

People have reported to me that, at the National Institutes of Health, patients are not given hospital gowns. They bring their own clothes, they make their own beds when possible, and they are given instruction about their own treatment. When they leave the hospital, they can take care of themselves because they have not been infantalized. At the Planetree Model Hospital Unit in San Francisco, patients wear their own clothes, sleep on flowered sheets, and can write in their own charts if they choose. Patients' relatives can visit whenever it's convenient for the patient, can cook for their loved ones in a special family kitchen, and learn to change dressings and tend to IV tubes if they choose. This way, they already know what to do when the patient comes home. Similar programs are in place at the Commonweal Cancer Help Program in Bolinas, California, and information about other programs is available from the American Self-Help Clearinghouse, in Denville, New Jersey. Dr. Michael Lerner, co-founder of the Commonweal Cancer Help Program, believes there are different levels of healing: biological, mental, and spiritual. Patients at Commonweal are guided in finding out what they can do to change their quality of life, and their relationship to their disease. The goal is to teach them stress reduction, health promotion, and group support. Stress reduction involves meditation, yoga, progressive deep relaxation, stretching, and massage. Connections between the mind and the body are explored during patients' one-week retreat.[2]

In most hospital situations, patients wear identical gowns and, to those caring for them, all look alike and seem alike. They are "Mrs. Jones with the kidney stone." They are not *people* with relationships. No one much cares what they ate or what lifestyle they lived before they came in. We operate and send them home quickly, and expect them to take immediate care of themselves. We put them in a dependent position, and expect them to be independent again with very little transition time, or time to heal from the trauma of surgery. In a system of sovereign practitioners and powerless patients, it's no wonder fear keeps people away. Certainly, the time to change this is now.

Cooperative Medicine

The combination of modern medical science and ancient techniques is the most powerful assortment humans have ever had at their disposal in the course of history. The breadth of techniques and information available to us in this century is truly astonishing. The relationship between modern scientists and traditional practitioners need not be adversarial. As consumers of varied medical therapies, we can demand that it not be adversarial. We can insist upon *cooperative medicine,* a combination approach to any medical problem. The peaceful confluence of philosophies is up to us, because it is we who ultimately pay. We need not permit divergence of professional opinions to *cost us our choices.* Loss of choice is most detrimental to the health of consumers. If we can utilize the best of both approaches, our quality of health and life can be improved. *At the behest of consumers,* more and more conventional institutions are now beginning to cull traditional ideas within their quest to diminish health care costs. For example, Dr. Andrew Weil, a long-time advocate of holistic health, has been appointed director of the University of Arizona Medical School's new Center for Integrated Healing, the first post-graduate program training doctors in alternative medicine in the United States.[3]

Holistic health care has, in the past, had a bad image. The public has been soured on nonconventional approaches by snake oil peddlers, shifty-eyed gurus, quacks, charlatans, and all manner of transcendental trippers. As holism becomes steeped in medical and health science evidence, however, such a negative image is changing. Holism offers a library of serious techniques that have worked for real people and are deserving of public attention.

We have covered a great deal of information in this book, but there is a lot more out there, and ongoing research changes what we know all the time. No one practitioner or researcher has all the answers. Health care becomes a way of thinking, of finding what your own individual belief system is and what works for you. Illness makes us ask, "How do I heal myself?" It's all there within us. We have to figure out how to tap into our *inner* as well as our outer resources. It has become important for us as practitioners to involve all our resources to find answers. I've been in health care for over 30 years. Along the way, everybody gave me one piece of information that I did not have before.

We need to know what questions to ask. Often when patients come to my office, they don't know what questions to ask. They're scared, and they fear the worst. This is particularly true in my practice, because women are intimidated by a gynecological exam. In response, I have tried to make them feel safe and comfortable, and this has taught me something. I may not be the teacher; rather, I may be the student. I used to think I was good at diagnosing because of my training and intuition, but now I believe that I am a truly good listener. I listen to patients, and I am not as threatened by that as I used to be. I used to think that I had to have gallons of data and laboratory tests, but now I know that's not always helpful. Patients come to me because they know my philosophy is that we will work together, as a team, to return balance to their bodies.

I encourage women to leave an office if they don't feel comfortable with the medical practitioner. Sometimes you can just feel things that aren't right—intuition, body responses, auras, or whatever you choose to call them. This is holistic health care—paying attention to what is going on, listening to yourself and your own body responses, and thinking about what you can do to make yourself well.

The way I see it, mind, body, and spirit form a trilogy. They are inseparable, all connected, and when we get sick, we need to know that they are all connected.

There are a variety of techniques available to heal the mind, body, and spirit. Only you know what will work for you. If I say, "Go get acupuncture," but you are frightened of needles, that will not work for you. You'll be tense, anxious, and your very cells will be locked up so securely you can feel it. You'll experience a stress response and the immune system will be affected. We need to be aware of our individual body's responses. If someone suggests something, what is your body's reaction? If anyone tells you, "This is the only way to do it," then you'd better run the other way. We don't know the "only" way. Nobody does. Only you know for you.

Each of us has a healer within that is activated when we need it. If you get diagnosed with a serious illness, you at first experience the sympathetic nervous response—you might feel dizzy, faint, scared, or have a loudly pounding heart. You're frightened and wondering what you're going to do, how you're going to cope. Once you can calm down, it is easier to feel that there is a healer within. How we get to that healer is an individual path. Yours is not like anyone else's.

Some practitioners look for metaphors of illness and try to help people discern what the symptom means. A patient once told me she had severe pain in her hand. As we talked, she realized she had to "handle" something that was frightening and challenging. Once she straightened out this difficulty in her life, her hand pain stopped. Pay attention to your body. It will tell you everything you need to know, and if you cannot figure it out yourself, seek out a health care practitioner who can help you get to that process, someone who will talk to you, touch you, help you get to that quiet state. These are powerful forces that we, in conventional medicine, cannot ignore any longer.

Marlo Morgan is a physician who went to Australia to investigate medical practices among the Aborigines. She worked for a year with them and wrote a book about her experiences, *Mutant Message Down Under*.[4] The Aborigines told her they were going to give her an award for the work she had done. She dressed up for the occasion in a nice suit, high-heeled shoes, and jewelry, and waited to be picked up at her hotel. The tribesmen took her far from the hotel, sat her down in a circle of people, took her clothes and jewelry from her, and dressed her in a native cloth. They took her on a walking journey, a "walkabout," that lasted four months and was in fact her "award." She had no shampoo, soap, deodorant, or other amenities and learned to live a subsistence lifestyle. She endured a daunting and often harrowing transition. When the tribesmen killed an animal to eat, they utilized every single part of it, down to the last bone, for some purpose. Nothing was wasted. They talked out loud almost never, much less than people Dr. Morgan was used to, but they communicated often using what is called "mental telepathy." They were very much in touch with intuitive processes and sensibilities. One night, one of the men fell into a ravine and broke his leg. The bone was fractured and protruding from the skin. The other people got him up out of the rocks within minutes, and got his bone back under the skin. A healer woman and a medicine man gave him some herbs and sealed his wound with bark, and then put him to sleep for the night. Then they sat with him all night, touching him and talking softly to him. In the morning, he walked by himself. Morgan felt that she had witnessed these people help their fellow to find the healer within himself. We have all probably heard stories or read books about healers who affect physical changes in sick people using only their hands. Perhaps what Morgan had witnessed was the power of touch in the process of healing. When she eventually returned to civilization, she had one big question: *Who has the modern medicine—them or us?*

I was moved by this story because this is exactly how I view my job as a nurse—to help people to find their healer within.

I talk to many physicians who are frustrated with primary care and with how to heal people. We are all recognizing that we have to reach out to other areas in order to help people get well. Just ordering lab tests and surgery does not work. It's important that both patients and practitioners listen to the inner messages, because patients usually know what's wrong if you listen to them. I have never known a woman who didn't know when she was pregnant. I don't need to do a pregnancy test—I ask them if they think they are pregnant and they nod their heads in the affirmative. The test merely validates what they know they feel. Women also know when something is wrong with their bodies, but, unfortunately, we don't listen to our bodies and by the time we do, we're pretty sick. Many times you know before the lab test that something is wrong. You just need to reach out to some professional whom you know will help you to put your body back into balance.

Taking all these steps does not mean you'll be well the rest of your life. It's a choice you make about the quality of life that you'll have, so listen to yourself. You have all the answers.

Listen. . .

      To whom?

To yourself.

      I can't hear myself.

Shh. . .

Listen. . .

      To whom?

To yourself.

      No one will love me.

Shh. . .

Listen. . .

      To whom?

To yourself.

      What about others?

Shh. . .

Listen. . .

      To whom?

To yourself.

Do you scream?

      No, not in years:

      I have to again.

Go ahead.

      Will it be all right?

Yes . . . listen

      To whom?

To yourself.[5]

from *Peace, Love, and Healing*
Dr. Bernie Siegel

Conclusion

As a women's health care Nurse Practitioner and as a woman, I was motivated to write this book in an effort to bring information and choices to a wide range of individuals. I am dedicated to helping people find their truth and their path to wholeness. This book is based upon personal and professional experience. I do not claim anything more than what my training, experience, and research have taught me. The results of empirical research are currently being questioned, as they are expected to lead to the truth; we must continue to search for the truth through whatever modality sets us free. I am not a laboratory scientist, but rather a professional who is seeking the answers by asking the questions. I respect the fact that there is much controversy and discussion about what heals people.

Let us all find our healer within.

Notes

Chapter 2

1. M. Kemeny, G. Solomon, J. E. Morley, & T. L. Herbert, "Psychoneuroimmunology," in C. B. Nemeroff (Ed.), *Neuroendocrinology,* (Boca Raton, FL: CRC Press Inc., 1992), pp. 563–591.

2. G. F. Solomon, M. E. Kemeny, & L. Temoshok, "Psychoneuroimmunologic aspects of human immunodeficiency virus infection," in R. Ader, D. L. Felten, & N. Cohen (Eds.), *Psychoneuroimmunology II,* (Orlando: Academic Press, 1991); Margaret Kemeny, R. Duran, H. Weiner, B. Visscher, & J. Fahey, "Bereavement of partner and immune processes in HIV positive and negative homosexual men," Seventh International Conference on AIDS, Florence, Italy, June 1991; and Margaret Kemeny, R. Duran, S. Taylor, H. Weiner, B. Visscher, & J. Fahey, "Chronic depression predicts CD4 decline over a five-year period in HIV seropositive men," Sixth International Conference on AIDS, San Francisco, June 1990.

3. Margaret Kemeny, & George Solomon, "Psychoneuroimmunology," Seminar on PNI, Esalen Institute, Big Sur, CA, October 8–10, 1993; and A. Amkraut & George Solomon, "Stress and murine sarcoma virus (Moloney)-induced tumors, *Cancer Research, 1428,* (1992), 32.

4. Deepak Chopra, *Ageless body, timeless mind,* (New York: Random House, 1993); *Perfect health,* (New York: Harmony Books, 1991), and *Creating health,* (Boston: Houghton Mifflin, 1991).

5. Robert Ornstein, & David Sobel, *The healing brain,* (New York: Simon & Schuster, 1987); Leonard White, Bernard Tursky, & Gary E. Schwarz, (Eds.), *Placebo: Theory, research, and mechanisms,* (New York: Guilford Press, 1985)); and Arthur K. Shapiro & L. A. Morris, "The placebo effect in medical and psychological

theories," in S. L. Garfield & A. E. Bergin (Eds.) *The handbook of psychotherapy and behavior change,* (New York: John Wiley, 1978).

6. Margaret Kemeny & George Solomon, "Psychoneuroimmunology," PNI Seminar at Esalen Institute, Big Sur, CA, October 8–10, 1993.

7. Steven Locke, & Douglas Colligan *The healer within* (New York: E. P. Dutton, 1987), p. 33.

8. Interview with Dr. Candace Pert in Betty S. Flowers, (Ed.), *Bill Moyers' healing and the mind,* (New York: Doubleday, 1993), pp. 177–193, companion publication to *Healing and the mind,* Bill Moyers, (Narr.) David Grubin Productions Inc., (Prod.) 1993, aired on PBS Television in 1993/94.

9. Dr. David Eisenberg, "Medicine in a mind/body culture," in Flowers, pp. 257–271. Eisenberg trained at a hospital in China where Chinese and Western medicine are both utilized, and he spoke with a woman whose fibrocystic breast pain was eliminated by a skilled massage doctor. For many years, she had sought relief from more conventional treatments and medications, to no avail.

10. Laura Norman with Thomas Cowan, *Feet first: A guide to foot reflexology* (New York: Simon & Schuster, 1988), p. 18.

11. Charles L. Votaw, "Morphology of the nervous system as related to trauma," in Stanley H. Backaitis, *Biomechanics of impact injury and injury tolerances of the head-neck complex* (Warrendale, PA: Society of Automotive Engineers, 1993), pp. 27–39; Jeffrey A. Pike, *Automotive safety: Anatomy, injury, testing, and regulations,* (Warrendale, PA: Society of Automotive Engineers, 1990).

Chapter 3

1. Carlton Fredericks, *The new low blood sugar and you* (New York: Putnam, 1985), pp. 117–119.

2. Biology and Neuroscience Professor Robert Sapolsky's book, *Why zebras don't get ulcers: A guide to stress, stress-related diseases, and coping* (New York: Freeman, 1994) includes citations of over 200

studies published in academic journals, suggesting causative links between stress and illness. Reviews of the various and historically opposing points of view concerning the connection between stress and illness can be found in J. P. Henry & P. M. Stephens, *Stress, health, and the social environment* (New York: Springer-Verlag, 1977); H. Weiner, *Psychobiology and human disease* (New York: American Elsevier, 1977); J. Cassel, "Psychosocial processes and 'stress': Theoretical formulation," *International Journal of Health Services, 4,* 1974, pp. 471–482; and Jerome David Frank, *Persuasion and healing* (Baltimore: Johns Hopkins Press, 1961). The early, ground-breaking research in this field is generally attributed to Cannon and Selye, found in Walter Cannon, "The role of emotion in disease," *Annals of Internal Medicine, 9:2,* May 1936, and Hans Selye, *The stress of my Life* (New York: Von Nostrand, 1979).

3. Sapolsky, p. 11.

4. Robert M. Rose, "Psychoendocrinology," in Jean D. Wilson, M.D., & Daniel W. Foster, M.D., (Eds.), *Textbook of endocrinology* (Philadelphia: Saunders, 1985), pp. 653–681.

5. S. J. Quinn & G. H. Williams, "Regulation of aldosterone secretion," *Annual Review of Physiology, 50:*409, 1988; G. P. Chrousos, T. H. Schuermeyer, J. Doppman, et al., "Clinical applications of corticotropin-releasing factor," *Annals of Internal Medicine,* 102:344, 1985; and D. N. Orth, "Corticotropin-releasing hormone in humans," *Endocrine Review, 13:*164, 1992.

6. Daniel D. Federman, "Endocrinology: The adrenal gland" in Edward Rubenstein, M.D., M.A.C.P., & Daniel D. Federman, M.D., M.A.C.P., (Eds.), *Scientific American Medicine* (New York: Scientific American Inc., 1994).

7. Fredericks, p. 28.

8. Fredericks, p. 91.

9. Fredericks.

'10. Fredericks, p. 91.

11. Fredericks, p. 95.

12. Dolores Krieger, *Accepting your power to heal: The personal practice of therapeutic touch* (Santa Fe: Bear and Co., 1993).

13. Steven Locke, & Douglas Colligan, *The healer within* (New York: E. P. Dutton, 1986), pp. 230–231.

14. Marie Cargill, *Acupuncture: A Viable Medical Alternative* (Westport, CT: Praeger Publishers, 1994); Mark Duke, *Acupuncture* (New York: Pyramid House Books, 1972).

15. B.K.S. Iyengar, *Light on yoga* (New York: Schocken Books, 1979).

16. Jon Kabat Zinn, *Wherever you go, there you are* (New York: Hyperion Books, 1994); *Full catastrophe living: Using the wisdom of your body and mind to face stress* (New York: Delacorte Press, 1990).

17. Andrew Weil, M.D. *Natural health, natural medicine* (Boston: Houghton Mifflin, 1990) pp. 83–90.

18. Margaret Kemeny & George Solomon, "Psychoneuroimmunology," Seminar on PNI, Esalen Institute, Big Sur, CA., October 8–10, 1993.

19. Norman Cousins, *Anatomy of an illness as perceived by the patient: Reflections on healing and regeneration* (New York: Norton Books, 1979); *Head first: The biology of hope and the healing power of the human spirit* (New York: Viking Penguin Books, 1990); Anne Wilson Schaef, *Laugh! I thought I'd die (if I didn't)* (New York: Ballantine Books, 1990).

20. Nicholas P. Plotnikoff, Robert E. Faith, Anthony J. Murgo, & Robert A. Good, (Eds.) *Enkephalins and endorphins, stress and the immune system* (New York: Plenum Press, 1986).

21. Steven Locke & Mady Horning-Rohann, (Eds.), *Mind and immunity: Behavioral immunology* (New York: Institute for the Advancement of Health, 1983).

22. Dr. David Spiegel, Professor of Psychiatry and Behavioral Sciences, and Director of the Psychosocial Treatment Laboratory at Stanford University School of Medicine, completed a study of the effects of support groups on breast cancer patients in 1989, and discussed the results with Bill Moyers in *Healing and the mind,* Betty S. Flowers, (Ed.), (New York: Doubleday, 1993), pp. 157–170, companion piece to *Healing and the mind,* (Narr.) David Grubin Productions Inc., (Prod.) Bill Moyers, 1993, aired on PBS Television in 1994.

23. Dr. Michael Lerner, founder and President of Commonweal, a health and environmental research center in Bolinas CA, and co-founder of the Commonweal Cancer Help Program, is a Fellow of the Fetzer Institute and a Policy Fellow of the Institute of Health

Policy Studies at the University of California, San Francisco, Medical School and a recognized authority in the field of unconventional cancer treatments. He spoke with Bill Moyers in *Healing and the mind,* Betty S. Flowers, (Ed.) (New York: Doubleday, 1993), companion piece to the television series.

24. Kemeny and Solomon at Esalen.

25. Carl O. Simonton & Reid Henson, with Brenda Hampton, *The healing journey* (New York: Bantam Books, 1992), and Stephanie Matthews Simonton & James L. Creighton, *Getting well again: A step-by-step self-help guide to overcoming cancer* (Los Angeles: J. P. Tarcher, 1978).

26. Benton Goldberg Group, (Eds.) *Alternative medicine: The definitive guide* (Puyallup, WA: Future Medicine Publishing Inc., 1993); Michael Murray & Joseph Pizzorno, *Encyclopedia of natural medicine* (Rocklin, CA: Prima Publishers, 1991).

27. Locke and Colligan, p. 95.

28. Sapolsky.

Chapter 4

1. Joan Borysenko, & Myroslav Borysenko, *The power of the mind to heal* (Carson, CA: Hay House, 1994).

2. Dr. Joseph Feinberg in Manhasset, N.Y.

3. Melody Beattie, *Codependent no more: How to stop controlling others and caring for yourself,* (Center City, MN: Hazelden Books, 1987), and *Beyond codependency: And getting better all the time* (San Francisco: Harper, 1989); Pia Mellody, *Breaking free: A recovery workbook for facing codependence* (San Francisco: Harper & Row, 1989), and *Facing codependence:What it is, where it comes from, how it sabotages our lives* (San Francisco: Perennial Library, 1989); and Anne Wilson Schaef, *Codependence: Misunderstood— mistreated* (San Francisco: Harper, 1992).

4. Louise Hay, *The power is within you* (Santa Monica: Hay House, 1991), and *You can heal your life* (Santa Monica: Hay House, 1987).

5. Carol Gilligan, *A different voice: Psychological theory and women's development* (Cambridge, MA: Harvard University Press, 1982).

6. Beattie.

7. Christiane Northrup, *Women's bodies, women's wisdom* (New York: Bantam Books, 1994), p. 217.

8. Northrup; and Deepak Chopra, *Ageless body, timeless mind* (New York: Random House, 1993), *Perfect health* (New York: Harmony Books, 1991), and *Creating health* (Boston: Houghton Mifflin, 1991).

9. F. G. Giustini, M.D. *Understanding hysterectomy* (New York: Walker and Co., 1979).

10. Northrup, pp. 73–76.

11. Ken Pelletier, *Mind as healer, mind as slayer* (New York: Delacorte Press, 1977), pp. 134–149; A. Justice, "Review of the effects of stress on cancer in laboratory animals: Importance of time of stress application and type of tumor." *Psychological Bulletin, 98,* (1985), 108; F. I. Fawzy, M. E. Kemeny, N. W. Fawzy, R. Elashoff, D. Morton, N. Cousins, & J. L. Fahey, "A structured psychiatric intervention for cancer patients. II. Changes over time in immunological parameters," *Archives of General Psychiatry, 729,* (1990), 47: S. M. Levy, R. B. Herberman, A. M. Maluish, B. Schlien, & M. Lippman, "Prognostic risk assessment in primary breast cancer by behavioral and immunological parameters," *Health Psychology, 4,* (1985) 99; S. Levy, R. Herberman, M. Lippman, & T. d'Angelo, "Correlation of stress factors with sustained depression of natural killer cell activity and predicted prognosis in patients with breast cancer," *Journal of Clinical Oncology, 5,* (1987), 348.

12. Northrup, p. 287.

13. Bobbie Aqua, Licensed Acupuncturist and Chinese Herbalist, "Breast health workshop," Women's Resources Office, Sag Harbor, New York, October 1994.

14. Steven Locke & Douglas Colligan, *The healer within* (New York: E. P. Dutton, 1987).

15. Borysenko & Borysenko.

Chapter 5

1. Christiane Northrup, *Women's bodies, women's wisdom* (New York: Bantam Books, 1994).

2. Steven Locke and Douglas Colligan, *The healer within*, (New York: E. F. Dutton, 1987), pp. 152–153.

3. Louise Hay, *The power within you* (Santa Monica: Hay House, 1991), and *You can heal your life* (Santa Monica: Hay House, 1987).

4. Susan Love, *Dr. Susan Love's breast book* (Boston: Addison-Wesley Publishing Co., 1990).

5. Deepak Chopra, *Ageless Body, Timeless Mind* (New York: Random House, 1993), *Perfect health* (New York: Harmony Books, 1991), and *Creating Health* (Boston: Houghton Mifflin, 1991); and Larry Dossey, M.D. *The power of prayer and the practice of medicine* (San Francisco: Harper, 1993).

6. Michael Castleman, "Doctors Aren't Detecting Cancer in Time," *Redbook*, October 1986, pp. 138–139, 218–222.

7. Irving Ariel, *Breast surgery, diagnosis and treatment* (New York: McGraw Hill Book Co., 1987), p. 205.

8. Henry P. Leis, Frederick L. Greene, J. Carlisle Hewitt, and James L. Haynes, "The War On Breast Cancer: Prevention and Early Detection," *The Female Patient*, 13, August 1988, pp. 57–62.

9. Love; and Delia Marshall, "Mammograms under 50," *Working Woman*, Vol. 19, October 10, 1994, pp. 41–43.

10. Love, pp. 181–182.

11. Jane Brody, "Some Radiologists Say Evidence Will Emerge in Time," *New York Times*, Sec. C, December 14, 1993, p. 1.

12. Patricia P. Kelly, Ph.D. *Understanding breast cancer risk* (Philadelphia: Temple University Press, 1991).

13. Love, p. 6.

14. Leis.

15. Bobbie Aqua, Licensed Acupuncturist and Chinese Herbalist, "Breast Cancer Seminar," Women's Resources Office, Sag Harbor, NY, October 1994.

16. Aqua.

17. Chopra.

18. Harriet Goldhor Lerner, *Dance of anger* (New York: Harper Collins, 1989).

19. Love, p. 152.

20. Jay M. Gould and Benjamin A. Goldman with Kate Millpointer, *Deadly deceit* (New York: Four Walls Eight Windows, 1990).

21. Christiane Northrup, M.D., "How to create breast health," *Creating Health Newsletter,* Vol. 3, Winter 1994; Allan Luks and Joseph Barbato, *You are what you drink* (New York: Villard Books, 1989), pp. 58–78; Matthew Longnecker, "A meta-analysis of alcohol consumption in relation to risk of breast cancer." *Journal of the American Medical Association,* August 5, 1988, 652–656; Arthur Schatzin, "Alcohol consumption and breast cancer in the epidemiologic follow-up study of the first national health and nutrition examination survey," *The New England Journal of Medicine,* 316, 19, May 7, 1987, 1169–1173; W. C. Willett, "Moderate alcohol consumption and the risk of breast cancer." *The New England Journal of Medicine,* 316, 19, May 7, 1987, 1174–1179.

22. Luks and Barbato, pp. 58–62.

23. Carlton Frederick, *The new low blood sugar and you* (New York: Putnam Publishing Group, 1985); Christiane Northrup, Newsletter.

24. Lynne Walker and Ellen Brown, *Breezing through the change* (Berkeley, CA: Frog Ltd., 1994), p. 122.

25. Jon J. Michnovicz, and Diane S. Klein, *How to reduce your risk of breast cancer* (New York: Warner Books, 1994), p. 117.

26. Lavon J. Dunne, *Nutrition almanac* (New York: McGraw Hill, 1990), pp. 60–62.

27. Michnovicz and Klein, pp. 109–110.

28. Northrup Newsletter.

29. Northrup, *Women's bodies, women's wisdom,* p. 296.

30. Love.

Chapter 6

1. Personal interview with Debby Kuriloff, Ph.D. and Sex Therapist, September 1992.

2. Kristen Von Kreisler, "Sexual healing," *Redbook,* April 1993, pp. 86–129.

3. Judith Sachs, *The healing power of sex.* (Englewood Cliffs, NJ: Prentice-Hall, 1991).

4. Reed Moskowitz, *Your healing mind* (New York: Morrow, 1992).

5. Winnifred Cutler, Ph.D., *Love cycles: The science of intimacy* (New York: Villard Books, 1991), p. 22. Cutler, a research biologist, is founder of the Athena Institute for Women's Wellness in Haverford, PA.

6. Cutler, p. 22.

7. Cutler, p. 19.

8. Sachs.

9. Abraham Maslow, *Toward a psychology of being* (New York: D. Van Nostrand, Co., 1968).

10. Michael Carrera, *The language of sex: An A To Z guide* (New York: Facts On File Inc., 1991).

11. Joan Borysenko, *Guilt is the teacher, love is the lesson* (New York: Warner Books, 1990).

12. Steven Locke & Douglas Colligan, *The healer within* (New York: E. P. Dutton, 1986), p. 147.

13. Christiane Northrup, M.D., *Women's bodies, women's wisdom* (New York: Bantam Books, 1994), pp. 259–261.

14. Allan Luks & Joseph Barbato, *You are what you drink* (New York: Villard Books, 1989), pp. 57–102; Robert Sapolsky, *Why zebras don't get ulcers: A guide to stress, stress-related diseases and coping* (New York: W. H. Freeman, 1994).

15. Sachs.

Chapter 7

1. Katarina Dalton, M.D., *The menstrual cycle* (New York: Pantheon Books, 1969).

2. Rollin McCraty's findings were presented at the International Montreux Congress on Stress in Montreux, Switzerland, March 1995, and at the American Psychosomatic Society in April 1995; Jamie Talan, "It's true—less stress soothes body and soul," *Newsday,* March 7, 1995, Sec. B, p. 36.

3. Susan Lark, *Pre-menstrual syndrome self-help book* (New York: Forman Publishing, 1984); Ann Nazzaro, *The PMS solution* (Minneapolis: Winston Press, 1985); Ronald Norris, *PMS: Premenstrual syndrome* (New York: Rawson Associates, 1983).

4. Carlton Frederick, *The new low blood sugar and you* (New York: Putman, 1985); Allan Luks & Joseph Barbato, *You are what you drink* (New York: Villard Books, 1989); Katherine Ketcham & L. Ann Mueller, M.D., *Eating right to live sober* (New York: Signet, 1983).

5. Niels H. Lauersen, M.D., & Eileen Stukare, *Pre-menstrual syndrome and you* (New York: Simon & Schuster, 1983) pp. 64–65.

6. Lynne Walker, & Ellen Brown, *Breezing through the change* (Berkeley, CA: Frog Ltd., 1994).

7. Women's International Pharmacy, Madison, WI; J. C. Prior, "Progesterone as a bone trophic hormone," *Endocrine Reviews, 11:* 2, May 1990, pp. 386–396.

8. Marie Cargill, *Acupuncture: A viable medical alternative* (Westport, CT: Praeger Publishers, 1994); Mark Duke, *Acupuncture* (New York: Pyramid House Books, 1972).

9. Paula Weideger, *Menstruation and menopause: The physiology and psychology, the myth and the reality.* (New York: Alfred A. Knopf, 1976).

Chapter 8

1. Philip Sarel, M.D., *Sexual turning points* (New York: Macmillan, 1984).

2. John R. Lee, "Osteoporosis review," *International Clinical Nutrition Review, 10,* #3, July 1990, pp. 384–391.

3. Lynne Walker, & Ellen Brown, *Breezing through the change* (Berkeley, CA: Frog Ltd., 1994), p. 141.

4. Alan R. Gaby, M.D., *Preventing and reversing osteoporosis* (Rocklin, CA: Prima Publishing, 1994).

5. Andrew Weil, M.D., *Self-Healing Newsletter, 1,* Issue 1, October 1995.

6. Dr. William Castelli, director of the 35-year Framingham Heart Study in Massachusetts, the longest running study of heart disease in the United States, cited in Mark Fuerst, "The cholesterol that counts," *American Health,* June 1992, pp. 77–78.

7. Betty Friedan, *The fountain of age* (New York: Simon & Schuster, 1993), pp. 472–499; Christiane Northrup, *Women's bod-*

ies, women's wisdom (New York, Bantam Books, 1994), "The medicalization of menopause has been very successful." p. 465.

8. Lonnie Barbach, *The pause: A positive approach to menopause* (New York: Dutton, 1993); Sadja Greenwood, *Menopause naturally* (Volcano, CA: Volcano Press, 1992); Utian H. Wulf and Ruth S. Jacobowitz, *Managing your Menopause* (New York: Simon and Schuster, 1991); Susan Lark, *The menopause self-help book* (Berkeley, CA: Celestial Arts, 1990); Penny Wise Budoff, *No more hot flashes and other good news* (New York: Putnam, 1983).

9. Walker & Brown, pp. 122–130.

10. Susun Weed, *Menopausal years* (Woodstock, NY: Ash Tree Publications, 1992).

11. Walker & Brown.

12. Marie Cargill, Acupuncture: A viable medical alternative (Westport, CT: Praeger, 1994); Mark Duke, *Acupuncture* (New York: Pyramid House Books, 1972).

13. Ann Louise Gittleman, *Super nutrition for menopause* (New York: Pocket Books, 1993).

14. Walker, & Brown, p. 122.

15. Gaby; and Gail Sheehy, *The silent passage* (New York: Random House, 1991), p. 110.

16. Sheehy, p. 111.

17. Lark; and Lynn Murray Willeford, "Menopause naturally," *New Age Journal,* September/October 1995, pp. 151–152.

18. The Women's International Pharmacy Company is located in Madison, WI.

19. Lila Nachtigall, & Joan R. Heilman, *Estrogen: A complete guide to reversing the effects of menopause using hormone replacement therapy* (New York: HarperCollins, 1991).

20. The postmenopausal estrogen/progesterone interventions trial (PEPI), conducted by the National Heart, Lung, and Blood Institute at the National Institutes for Health, results released November 17, 1994.

21. Walker & Brown, p. 25.

22. Christiane Northrup, *Women's bodies, women's wisdom,* (New York: Bantam Books, 1994), p. 467.

23. John Lee.

24. Willeford.
25. Margaret Mead, *Male and female* (New York: William Morrow, 1949), pp. 368–384; and Friedan, p. 499.

Chapter 9

1. John P. Bradley, Leo F. Daniels, and Thomas C. Jones, *The International Dictionary of Thought* (Chicago: J. P. Ferguson, 1969), p. 720.
2. Dean Ornish, *Dr. Dean Ornish's program for reversing heart disease* (Ballantine Books, 1990).
3. Robert Pritikin, *The new Pritikin program,* (New York: Simon & Schuster, 1990); Nathan Pritikin with Patrick Grady, *The Pritikin program for diet and exercise* (New York: Grosset and Dunlop, 1979).
4. Deepak Chopra speaking at The Learning Annex, New York City, March 1994.
5. John Robbins, *Diet for a new America* (Walpole, NH: Stillpoint Publishers, 1987).
6. Artemis Simopoulos, M.D., Victor Herbert, M.D., J. D., & Beverly Jacobson, *Genetic nutrition* (New York: Macmillan Co., 1993), pp. 5–6, 198, 200.
7. William Dufty, *Sugar blues,* (New York: Warner Books, 1986).
8. William G. Crook, M.D., *The yeast connection* (Jackson, TN: Professional Books/Future Health Inc., 1985).
9. Susan Lark, M.D., *The menopause self-help book* (Berkeley, CA: Celestial Arts, 1990); Lynn Murray Willeford, "Menopause naturally," *New Age Journal,* September/October 1995, pp. 151–152.
10. Linda G. Rector-Page, *Healthy healing* (Sierra Foothills, CA: Healthy Healing Publications, 1994), p. 19; James F. Balch, M.D., & Phyllis A. Balch, C.N.C., *Prescriptions for nutritional healing* (Garden City, NY: Avery Publishing Group Inc., 1990), pp. 9–10.
11. Bernie Siegel, M.D., *Love, medicine, and miracles* (New York: HarperCollins, 1990).
12. Joan Borysenko, *Fire in the soul: A new psychology of spiritual optimism* (New York: Warner Books, 1993), *Guilt is the teacher, love is the lesson* (New York: Warner Books, 1990), *Minding the*

body, mending the mind (Reading, MA: Addison-Wesley Publishing Co., 1987) and co-author with Myroslav Borysenko, *The power of the mind to heal* (Carson, CA: Hay House, 1994).

Chapter 10

1. I generally recommend the books listed in the bibliography.

2. Dr. Michael Lerner speaking in Betty S. Flowers, (Ed.) *Bill Moyers healing and the mind* (New York: Doubleday, 1993), p. 323, companion piece to *Healing and the mind,* Bill Moyers, (Narr.) David Grubin Productions, Inc., (Prod.) 1993, aired on PBS Television in 1994.

3. Andrew Weil, M.D., & Bernie Siegal, M.D., "Complimentary medicines," Body and Soul II Conference, Boston, MA, September 15–17, 1995; Andrew Weil, M.D., *Natural health, natural medicine* (Boston: Houghton Mifflin, 1990), and *Health and healing* (Boston: Houghton Mifflin, 1983).

4. Marlo Morgan, *Mutant message down under* (New York: HarperCollins, 1994).

5. Bernie Siegal, M.D., *Love, medicine, and miracles* (New York: HarperCollins, 1990).

Bibliography

Psychoneuroimmunology

Books and Articles

Borysenko, Joan & Myroslav Borysenko. *The Power of the Mind to Heal.* Carson, CA: Hay House, 1994.

_____. *Fire in the Soul: A New Psychology of Spiritual Optimism.* New York: Warner Books, 1993.

_____. *Guilt is the Teacher, Love Is the Lesson.* New York: Warner Books, 1990.

_____. *Minding the Body, Mending the Mind.* Reading, MA: Addison-Wesley, 1987.

Brennan, Barbara. *Hands of Light.* New York: Bantam, 1988.

Chopra, Deepak. *Ageless Body: Timeless Mind.* New York: Random House, 1993.

_____. *Perfect Health.* New York: Harmony Books, 1989.

_____. *Creating Health.* Boston: Houghton Mifflin, 1987.

Cousins, Norman. *Head First: The Biology of Hope and the Healing Power of the Human Spirit.* New York: Viking Penguin, 1990.

_____. *Anatomy of an Illness: Reflections on Healing and Regeneration.* New York: Norton Books, 1979.

Damasio, Antonio. *Descartes' Error: Emotion, Reason and the Human Brain.* New York: Putnam, 1995.

Dienstfrey, Harris. *Where the Mind Meets the Body.* New York: Harper Collins, 1991.

Dossey, Larry. *Healing Words: The Power of Prayer and the Practice of Medicine.* San Francisco: Harper, 1993.

Flowers, Betty S. (Ed.). *Bill Moyers' Healing and the Mind.* New York: Doubleday, 1993. Companion piece to the video *Bill Moyers' Healing and the Mind.* Bill Moyers, (Narr.), David Grubin, (Prod.), PBS Television, 1994.

Hay, Louise L. *The Power Is within You.* Carson, CA: Hay House, 1991.

_____. *You Can Heal Your Life.* Carson, CA: Hay House, 1987.

Kabat-Zinn, Jon. *Wherever You Go, There You Are: Mindfulness Meditation in Everyday Life.* New York: Hyperion, 1994.

_____. *Full Catastrophe Living: Using the Wisdom of Your Body and Mind to Face Stress.* New York: Delacorte Press, 1990.

Linn, Amy. "When the Body Heals Itself." *Ladies' Home Journal,* May 1995, p. 118.

Locke, Steven & Douglas Colligan. *The Healer Within.* New York: Dutton, 1986.

Northrup, Christiane. *Women's Bodies, Women's Wisdom.* New York: Bantam Books, 1994.

Ornstein, Robert & David Sobel. *The Healing Brain.* New York: Simon and Schuster, 1988.

Rosenberg, Steven. *The Transformed Cell.* New York: Putnam, 1992.

Siegel, Bernie. *Love, Medicine, and Miracles.* New York: Harper Collins, 1990.

_____. *Peace, Love, and Healing: Bodymind Communication and the Path to Self-Healing.* New York: Harper Collins, 1990.

Academic Sources

Ader, Robert (Ed.). *Psychoneuroimmunology.* New York: Academic Press, 1981.

Bergsma, Daniel & Allan L. Goldstein (Eds.). *Neurochemical and Immunologic Components in Schizophrenia.* New York: Alan R. Liss, 1978.

Frederickson, Robert C. A., Hugh C. Hendrie, Jospeh N. Hingten, & Morris H. Aprison (Eds.). *Neuroregulation of Autonomic Endocrine and Immune Systems.* Boston: Martinus Nijhoff, 1986.

Kemeny, Margaret E., George F. Solomon, J. E. Morley, & T. L. Herbert. "Psychoneuroimmunology." In C. B. Nemeroff (Ed.), *Neuroendocrinology.* Boca Raton, FL: CRC Press, Inc., 1992.

Korneva, Elena A., Viktor M. Klimenko, & Elenora K. Shkhinek. *Maintenance of Immune Homeostasis.* Chicago: University Of Chicago Press, 1985.

Locke, Steven E. (Ed.). *Psychological and Behavioral Treatments for Disorders Associated with the Immune System: An Annotated Bibliography.* New York: Institute for the Advancement of Health, 1986.

———, Robert Ader, Hugo Besedovsky, Nicholas Hall, George Solomon, & Terry Strom (Eds.). *Foundations of Psychoneuroimmunology.* New York: Aldine, 1985.

———, & Mady Horning-Rohann (Eds.). *Mind and Immunity: Behavioral Immunology, an Annotated Bibliography.* New York: Institute for the Advancement of Health, 1983.

White, Leonard, Bernard Tursky, & Gary E. Schwarz (Eds.). *Placebo: Theory, Research, and Mechanisms.* New York: Guilford Press, 1985.

Young, Stuart H., James M. Rubin, & Harlan R. Daman (Eds.). *Psychobiological Aspects of Allergic Disorders.* New York: Praeger, 1986.

Stress and Its Effects

Books and Articles

Pelletier, Ken. *Holistic Medicine: From Stress to Optimal Health.* New York: Delacorte Press, 1979.

Sapolsky, Robert M. *Why Zebras Don't Get Ulcers: A Guide to Stress, Stress-Related Disease, and Coping.* New York: W. H. Freeman Co., 1994.

Academic Sources

Cooper, Edwin L. (Ed.). *Stress, Immunity, and Aging.* New York: Dekker, 1984.

Plotnikoff, Nicholas P., Robert E. Faith, Anthony J. Murgo, & Robert A. Good (Eds.). *Enkephalins and Endorphins, Stress and the Immune System.* New York: Institute for the Advancement of Health, 1983.

Codependency and Illness

Beattie, Melody. *A Reason to Live*. Wheaton, IL: Tyndale House, 1991.

_____. *Codependent's Guide to the Twelve Steps*. New York: Prentice-Hall Parkside, 1990.

_____. *The Language of Letting Go*. San Francisco: Harper & Row, 1990.

_____. *Beyond Codependency: And Getting Better All the Time*. San Francisco: Harper, 1989.

_____. *Codependent No More: How to Stop Controlling Others and Caring for Yourself*. Center City, MN: Hazelden, 1987.

Bradshaw, John. *Creating Love: The Next Stage of Growth*. New York: Bantam Books, 1992.

_____. *Homecoming: Reclaiming and Championing Your Inner Child*. New York: Bantam Books, 1990.

_____. *Bradshaw On: The Family*. Deerfield Beach, FL: Health Communications, 1988.

_____. *Healing the Shame That Binds You*. Deerfield Beach, FL: Health Communications, 1988.

Dowling, Collette. *You Mean I Don't Have to Feel This Way? New Help for Depression, Anxiety, Addiction*. New York: Scribner, 1991.

_____. *Perfect Women: Hidden Fears of Inadequacy and the Drive to Perform*. New York: Summit Books, 1988.

_____. *The Cinderella Complex*. New York: Summit Books, 1981.

Forward, Susan. *Obsessive Love: When It Hurts Too Much to Let Go*. New York: Bantam Books, 1992.

_____. *Toxic Parents: Overcoming Their Hurtful Legacy and Reclaiming Your Life*. New York: Bantam Books, 1989.

_____, & Craig Buck. *Betrayal of Innocence: Incest and Its Devastation*. New York: Penguin Books, 1987.

_____, & Joan Torres. *Men Who Hate Women and the Women Who Love Them*. New York: Bantam Books, 1986.

Mellody, Pia. *Facing Love Addiction: Giving Yourself the Power to Change the Way You Love*. San Francisco: Harper, 1992.

_____. *Breaking Free: A Recovery Workbook for Facing Codependence*. San Francisco: Harper & Row, 1989.

_____. *Facing Codependence: What It Is, Where It Comes From, How It Sabotages Our Lives.* San Francisco: Perennial Library, 1989.

Miller, Alice. *Breaking Down the Wall of Silence.* New York: Dutton, 1991.

_____. *The Drama of the Gifted Child.* New York: Basic Books, 1990.

_____. *Thou Shalt Not Be Aware.* New York: Farrar, Straus, Giroux, 1984.

_____. *For Your Own Good.* New York: Farrar, Straus, Giroux, 1983.

Norwood, Robin. *Women Who Love Too Much: When You Keep Wishing And Hoping He'll Change.* Los Angeles: J. P. Tarcher, 1985.

Schaef, Anne Wilson. *Beyond Therapy, Beyond Science: A New Model For Healing the Whole Person.* San Francisco: Harper, 1994.

_____. *Codependence: Misunderstood—Mistreated.* San Francisco: Harper, 1992.

_____. *Meditations for Women Who Do Too Much.* San Francisco: Harper, 1992.

_____. *Escape From Intimacy.* San Francisco: Harper & Row, 1990.

_____. *Laugh! I Thought I'd Die (If I Didn't).* New York: Ballantine Books, 1990.

_____. *Women's Reality: An Emerging Female System in a White Male Society.* San Francisco: Harper, 1985.

Woititz, Janet. *Adult Children of Alcoholics.* Deerfield, FL: Health Communications, 1983.

Breast Illness

Hunt, Diana. "Mammogram Alert." *East/West.* September/October 1991, p. 109.

Love, Susan. *Dr. Susan Love's Breast Book.* Reading, MA: Addison-Wesley, 1990.

Manes, Christopher. "The Cancer Legacy." *Lear's*, September 1993, p. 53.

Michnovicz, Jon J. & Diane S. Klein. *How to Reduce Your Risk of Breast Cancer.* New York: Warner Books, 1994.

Northrup, Christiane. "How to Create Breast Health." *Creating Health Newsletter,* Vol. 3, Winter 1994.

Sexuality and Sexually Transmitted Disease

Barbach, Lonnie. *For Yourself: The Fulfillment of Female Sexuality.* Garden City, NY: Doubleday, 1975.

Carnes, Patrick. *A Gentle Path Through the Twelve Steps.* Tucson: CompCare Publications, 1989.

_____. *Out of the Shadows: Understanding Sexual Addiction.* Tucson: CompCare Publications, 1985.

Carrera, Michael. *The Language of Sex: An A to Z Guide.* New York: Facts on File Inc., 1969.

Dodson, Betty. *Sex for One: The Joy of Self Loving.* New York: Harmony Books, 1987.

LoPiccolo, Joseph & Julia Heiman. *Becoming Orgasmic: A Sexual and Personal Growth Program for Women.* New York: Prentice-Hall, 1987.

Masters, William H., and Virginia E. Johnson, *Human Sexual Response.* Boston: Little Brown, 1966.

Sarel, Philip. *Sexual Turning Points.* New York: Macmillan, 1984.

Woititz, Janet. *Healing Your Sexual Self.* Deerfield Beach, FL: Health Communications, 1989.

PMS, Perimenopause, and Menopause

Books and Articles

Barbach, Lonnie. *The Pause: A Positive Approach to Menopause.* New York: Dutton, 1993.

Budoff, Penny Wise. *No More Hot Flashes and Other Good News.* New York: Putnam, 1983.

Dalton, Katarina. *The Menstrual Cycle.* New York: Pantheon Books, 1969.

Gaby, Alan R. *Preventing and Reversing Osteoporosis.* Rocklin, CA: Prima Publishing, 1994.

Gittleman, Ann Louise. *Super Nutrition for Menopause.* New York: Pocket Books, 1993.

Greenwood, Sadja. *Menopause Naturally.* Volcano, CA: Volcano Press, 1992.

Lark, Susan. *Menopause Self-Help Book.* Berkeley, CA: Celestial Arts, 1990.

_____. *Premenstrual Syndrome Self-Help Book.* New York: Forman Publishing, 1984.

Lauersen, Niels H. & Eileen Stukare. *Pre-Menstrual Syndrome and You.* New York: Simon and Schuster, 1983.

Nachtigall, Lila & Joan R. Heilman. *Estrogen: A Complete Guide to Reversing the Effects of Menopause Using Hormone Replacement Therapy.* New York: Harper Collins, 1991.

Nazzaro, Ann. *The PMS Solution.* Minneapolis: Winston Press, 1985.

Norris, Ronald V. *PMS/Premenstrual Syndrome.* New York: Rawson Associates, 1983.

Sheehy, Gail. *The Silent Passage.* New York: Random House, 1991.

Walker, Lynne & Ellen Brown. *Breezing Through the Change.* Berkeley, CA: Frog Ltd., 1994.

Weed, Susun. *Menopausal Years.* Woodstock, NY: Ash Tree Publications, 1992.

Willeford, Lynn Murray. "Menopause Naturally." *New Age Journal.* September/October 1995, pp. 151–152.

Wulf, Utian H. & Ruth S. Jacobowitz. *Managing Your Menopause.* New York: Simon and Schuster, 1991.

Academic Sources

Lee, John R. "Osteoporosis Review." *International Clinical Nutrition Review.* Vol. 10, #3, July 1990, pp. 384–391.

Prior, J. C. "Progesterone as a Bone Trophic Hormone." *Endocrine Reviews,* Vol. 11, May 1990, pp. 386–396.

Wellness and Psychology

Achterberg, Jeanne. *Imagery in Healing: Shamanism and Modern Medicine.* Boston: Shambhala, 1985.

American College of Sports Medicine. *ACSM Fitness Book.* Champaign, IL: Human Kinetics Publishers, 1992.

Andrews, Lynn. *Medicine Woman.* New York: Harper Paperbacks, 1991.

Ardell, Donald. *High Level Wellness.* Berkeley, CA: Ten Speed Press, 1986.

_____. *Fourteen Days to Wellness Lifestyle.* Mill Valley, CA: Whatever Publishers, 1982.

Asistent, Niro Markoff, with Paul Duffy. *Why I Survive AIDS.* New York: Fireside/Simon and Schuster, 1991.

Balch, James F. & Phyllis A. Balch. *Prescriptions for Nutritional Healing.* Garden City, NY: Avery Publishing Group, Inc., 1990.

Barnard, Neal D. *The Power of Your Plate: Eating Well for Better Health.* Summertown, TN: Book Publishing Company, 1990.

Benson, Herbert & Eileen Stuart. *The Wellness Book.* New York: Simon and Schuster, 1992.

_____. *Your Maximum Mind.* New York: New York Times Books, 1987.

_____, & Miriam Z. Klipper. *The Relaxation Response.* New York: William Morrow, 1975.

Benton Goldberg Group (Eds.). *Alternative Medicine, The Definitive Guide.* Puyallup, WA: Future Medicine Publishing, Inc., 1993.

Boston Women's Health Collective. *The New Our Bodies, Our Selves.* New York: Simon and Schuster, 1984.

Brown, Lyn Mikel & Carol Gilligan. *Meeting at the Crossroads: Women's Psychology and Girls' Development.* Cambridge, MA: Harvard University Press, 1992.

Cargill, Marie. *Acupuncture: A Viable Medical Alternative.* Westport, CT: Praeger Publishers, 1994

Castillejo, Irene Claremont. *Knowing Woman.* New York: Putnam Publications, 1973.

Cayce, Edgar. *The Edgar Cayce Collection, Vols. I–IV.* New York: Random House, 1986.

Crook, William G. *The Yeast Connection.* Jackson, TN: Professional Books/Future Health Inc., 1985.

Dufty, William. *Sugar Blues.* New York: Warner Books, 1986.

Duke, Mark. *Acupuncture.* New York: Pyramid House Books, 1972.

Dunne, Lavon J. *Nutrition Almanac, 3rd Ed.* New York: McGraw-Hill, 1990.

Estes, Clarissa Pinkola. *Women Who Run with the Wolves.* New York: Ballantine Books, 1994.

Ferguson, Tom. *Tom Ferguson's Health in the Information Age Letter* (quarterly), Self-Care Productions, 3805 Stevenson Ave., Austin, TX. 78703.

Frederick, Carlton. *The New Low Blood Sugar and You.* New York: Putnam Publishers, 1985.

Friedan, Betty. *The Fountain of Age.* New York: Simon and Schuster, 1993.

_____ . *The Second Stage.* New York: Summit Books, 1981.

_____ . *The Feminine Mystique.* New York: Norton Books, 1974.

Friedman, Meyer & Diane Ulmer. *Treating Type A Behavior and Your Heart.* New York: Fawcett, 1985.

Gawain, Shakti. *Creative Visualization.* New York: Bantam, 1983.

Gilligan, Carol. *Making Connections: The Relational Worlds of Adolescent Girls.* Cambridge, MA: Harvard University Press, 1989.

_____ . *A Different Voice.* Cambridge, MA: Harvard University Press, 1982.

_____ . *The Contribution Of Women's Thought To Developmental Theory.* Cambridge, MA: Harvard University Press, 1982.

Gittleman, Ann Louise & John M. Desgrey. *Beyond Pritikin.* New York: Bantam Books, 1989.

Goleman, Daniel & Joel Gurin (Eds.). *Mind Body Medicine: How to Use Your Mind for Better Health,* Consumer Reports Books, Consumers Union, 1993.

Iyengar, B. K. S. *Light on Yoga.* New York: Schocken Books, 1979.

Jaffe, Dennis T. *Healing from Within: Psychological Techniques to Help the Mind Heal the Body.* New York: Simon and Schuster, 1986.

Jung, Carl G. *Man and His Symbols.* New York: Doubleday, 1969.

Krieger, Dolores. *Accepting Your Power to Heal: The Personal Practice of Therapeutic Touch.* Santa Fe: Bear and Co., 1993.

Kurtz, Ernest & Katherine Ketcham. *The Spirituality of Imperfection.* New York: Bantam Books, 1992.

Lerner, Harriet Goldhor. *The Dance of Deception.* New York: Harper Collins, 1993.

_____. *The Dance of Intimacy.* Harper and Row, 1989.

_____. *The Dance of Anger.* New York: Perennial Library, 1989.

Leonard, Linda. *Meeting the Madwoman.* New York: Bantam Books, 1993.

_____. *Witness to the Fire: Creativity and the Veil of Addiction.* Boston: Shambhala, 1989.

_____. *On the Way to the Wedding.* Boston: Shambhala, 1987.

_____. *The Wounded Woman.* Athens, OH: Swallow Press, 1982.

Luks, Allan & Joseph Barbato. *You Are What You Drink.* New York: Villard Books, 1989.

Morgan, Marlo. *Mutant Message Down Under.* New York: Harper Collins, 1994.

Murray, Michael & Joseph Pizzorno. *Encyclopedia of Natural Medicine.* Rocklin, CA: Prima Publishers, 1991.

Northrup, Christiane. *Holistic Medicine: A Meeting of East And West.* Tokyo: Japan Publishing, 1992.

Ornish, Dean. *Dr. Dean Ornish's Program for Reversing Heart Disease.* New York: Ballantine Books, 1992.

Pelletier, Ken. *Healthy People in Unhealthy Places.* New York: Delacorte Press/Seymour Lawrence, 1984.

_____. *Mind as Healer, Mind as Slayer.* New York: Delacorte Press, 1977.

Pennebaker, James W. *Opening Up: The Healing Power of Confiding in Others.* New York: William Morris, 1990.

Pritikin, Robert. *The New Pritikin Program.* New York: Simon and Schuster, 1990.

Ray, Sondra. *I Deserve Love: How Affirmations Can Guide You to Personal Fulfillment.* Berkeley, CA: Celestial Arts, 1976.

Rector-Page, Linda G. *Healthy Healing.* Sierra Foothills, CA: Healthy Healing Publications, 1994.

Robbins, John. *Diet for a New America.* Walpole, NH: Stillpoint, 1987.

Rodegast, Pat & Judith Stanton. *Emmanuel's Book*. New York: Bantam Books, 1987.

Rossman, Martin. *Healing Yourself*. New York: Walker Publishing, 1987.

Sanuels, Michael. *Healing with the Mind's Eye*. New York: Random House, 1992.

Schlosberg, Suzanne. "Body Language—Moody? Depressed? Tired? Translation: You Could Be Getting the Word That Your Diet Is All Wrong." *Los Angeles Times*. Sec. E, October 3, 1995, pp. 1, 5.

Siegel, Bernie. *How to Live Between Office Visits*. New York: Harper Collins, 1993.

Simonton, O. Carl & Reid Henson, with Brenda Hampton. *The Healing Journey*. New York: Bantam Books, 1994.

_____, Stephanie Matthews Simonton & James L. Creighton. *Getting Well Again: A Step by Step Self Help Guide to Overcoming Cancer for Patients and Their Families*. Los Angeles: J. P. Tarcher, 1978.

Smith, John M. *Women and Doctors: A Physician's Explosive Account of Women's Medical Treatment*. New York: Atlantic Monthly Press, 1992.

Tavris, Carol. *Anger: The Misunderstood Emotion*. New York: Simon and Schuster, 1989.

Vuori, Ilkka. "Exercising for Health." *World Health Forum* (publication of the World Health Organization), 8, no. 2, 1982, pp. 131–140.

Weil, Andrew. *Natural Health, Natural Medicine*. Boston: Houghton Mifflin, 1990.

_____. *Health and Healing*. Boston: Houghton Mifflin, 1983.

Organizations and Resources

The Academy of Guided Imagery
P.O. Box 2070
Mill Valley, CA 94942
800-726-2070

Bibliography

American Association of Sex Educators, Counselors, and Therapists
435 N. Michigan Ave., Suite 1717
Chicago, IL 60611
312-644-0828

American Self-Help Clearinghouse
St. Clares—Riverside Medical Center
25 Pocono Road
Denville, NJ
201-625-7101

American Society of Clinical Hypnosis
2200 East Devon Ave., Suite 291
Des Plains, IL 60018

Awareness and Relaxation Training
Cabrillo College Stroke Center
501 Upper Park, De La Veago Park
Santa Cruz, CA 95065
408-722-9005

Biofeedback Certification Institute of America
10200 West 44th Ave., Suite 304
Wheatridge, CO 80033
303-420-2902

Cambridge Insight Meditation Center
331 Broadway
Cambridge, MA 02139
617-491-5070

The Fetzer Institute
9292 West KL Ave.
Kalamazoo, MI 49009
616-375-2000

Insight Meditation Society
Pleasant St.
Barre, MA 01005
508-355-4378

Insight Meditation West
P.O. Box 909
Woodacre, CA. 94973
415-488-0164

The Institute of Transpersonal Psychology
744 San Antonio Rd.
Palo Alto, CA 94303
415-493-4430

The Mind/Body Medical Institute, Division of Behavioral Medicine
New England Deaconess Hospital
185 Pilgrim Rd.
Boston, MA 02215
617-732-9530

The Society for Clinical and Experimental Hypnosis
128-A Kingspark Drive
Liverpool, NY 13090
315-652-7299

Stress Reduction Clinic
University of Massachusetts Medical Center
Worcester, MA 01655
508-856-1616

Index

About the Authors

Beth Moran, R.N., C.N.P., is a nurse practitioner who specializes in holistic and traditional health care for women. She is guest lecturer at SUNY Stony Brook and has appeared on *CBS This Morning*, *The McNeil Lehrer Report*, and *Medical News Network*. She is the founder and director of Women's Resources, Sag Harbor, New York, which she opened to give health care and health information to women, thus helping them make choices in their lives. She is also former director of Planned Parenthood, Riverhead, NY, and patient advocate/administrator of The New York Hospital. Beth Moran is a graduate of Pennsylvanuia Hospital, Margaret Sanger Center and Marymount Manhattan College.

Kathy Schultz is a freelance writer/researcher. She holds a B.A. in History from the University of Michigan and an M.S. in Psychology from Long Island University. In 1993–1995, she produced "Holistic Health Care with Beth Moran," a weekly broadcast for local television, and recently wrote and produced her first short film.